Surgery - Procedures, Complications, and Results

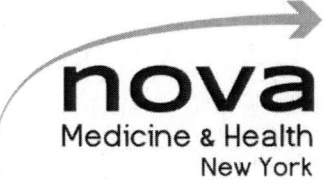

Surgery - Procedures, Complications, and Results

Nosocomial Infection in Abdominal Surgery
Jaime Ruiz-Tovar, MD, PhD (Editor)
Andrés García Marín, PhD (Editor)
2022. ISBN: 978-1-68507-603-0

Tracheostomy: Indications, Safety and Outcomes
Amit Agrawal, MD (Editor)
2022. ISBN: 978-1-68507-188-2 (Hardcover)
2021. ISBN: 978-1-68507-263-6 (eBook)

Enhanced Recovery after Surgery (ERAS) in Bariatric Surgery
Jaime Ruiz-Tovar, MD, PhD (Editor)
2021. ISBN: 978-1-53619-976-5 (Hardcover)
2021. ISBN: 978-1-68507-026-7 (eBook)

Enhanced Recovery After Surgery: Perspectives, Protocols and Efficacy
Stan Waechter (Editor)
2021. ISBN: 978-1-53619-548-4 (Softcover)
2021. ISBN: 978-1-53619-604-7 (eBook)

A Surgeon's Perspective on Dialysis Patients
Maria Frankovicova (Editor)
2021. ISBN: 978-1-53619-262-9 (Hardcover)
2021. ISBN: 978-1-53619-314-5 (eBook)

Encyclopedia of Surgery (22 Volume Set)
Andreas Lehrer and Kristin Mueller (Editors)
2020. ISBN: 978-1-53618-329-0 (Hardcover)
2020. ISBN: 978-1-53618-388-7 (eBook)

More information about this series can be found at
https://novapublishers.com/product-category/series/surgery-procedures-complications-and-results/

Jaime Ruiz-Tovar
and
Andrés García Marín
Editors

Nosocomial Infection in Abdominal Surgery

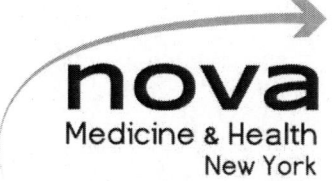

Copyright © 2022 by Nova Science Publishers, Inc.
DOI: https://doi.org/10.52305/HQVC9383

All rights reserved. No part of this book may be reproduced, stored in a retrieval system or transmitted in any form or by any means: electronic, electrostatic, magnetic, tape, mechanical photocopying, recording or otherwise without the written permission of the Publisher.

We have partnered with Copyright Clearance Center to make it easy for you to obtain permissions to reuse content from this publication. Simply navigate to this publication's page on Nova's website and locate the "Get Permission" button below the title description. This button is linked directly to the title's permission page on copyright.com. Alternatively, you can visit copyright.com and search by title, ISBN, or ISSN.

For further questions about using the service on copyright.com, please contact:
Copyright Clearance Center
Phone: +1-(978) 750-8400   Fax: +1-(978) 750-4470   E-mail: info@copyright.com.

NOTICE TO THE READER

The Publisher has taken reasonable care in the preparation of this book, but makes no expressed or implied warranty of any kind and assumes no responsibility for any errors or omissions. No liability is assumed for incidental or consequential damages in connection with or arising out of information contained in this book. The Publisher shall not be liable for any special, consequential, or exemplary damages resulting, in whole or in part, from the readers' use of, or reliance upon, this material. Any parts of this book based on government reports are so indicated and copyright is claimed for those parts to the extent applicable to compilations of such works.

Independent verification should be sought for any data, advice or recommendations contained in this book. In addition, no responsibility is assumed by the Publisher for any injury and/or damage to persons or property arising from any methods, products, instructions, ideas or otherwise contained in this publication.

This publication is designed to provide accurate and authoritative information with regard to the subject matter covered herein. It is sold with the clear understanding that the Publisher is not engaged in rendering legal or any other professional services. If legal or any other expert assistance is required, the services of a competent person should be sought. FROM A DECLARATION OF PARTICIPANTS JOINTLY ADOPTED BY A COMMITTEE OF THE AMERICAN BAR ASSOCIATION AND A COMMITTEE OF PUBLISHERS.

Additional color graphics may be available in the e-book version of this book.

Library of Congress Cataloging-in-Publication Data

ISBN: 978-1-68507-603-0

Published by Nova Science Publishers, Inc. † New York

Contents

Preface vii

Chapter 1 **Epidemiology of Nosocomial Infection** 1
José Ruiz Pardo and Clara Eugenia Cobo Cervantes

Chapter 2 **Risk Factors for Nosocomial Infection** 7
Francisco Javier Ruescas García
and Celia Pérez Parra

Chapter 3 **Prophylactic Measures against Surgical Site Infection after Abdominal Surgery** 19
Jaime Ruiz-Tovar

Chapter 4 **Microbiology and Treatment of Nosocomial Site Infection** 35
Andrés García Marín and Mercedes Pérez-López

Chapter 5 **Nosocomial Urinary Tract Infection** 45
Ana Sánchez-Mozo and Héctor Aguado-López

Chapter 6 **Nosocomial Respiratory Tract Infection** 59
Francisco Javier Ruescas García
and Celia Pérez Parra

Chapter 7 **Vascular Access Infection** 73
Héctor Aguado López and Ana Sánchez Mozo

Chapter 8 **Endocarditis and Intravascular Infections** 91
Covadonga Martín Garrido

Chapter 9 **Pseudomembranous Colitis and Other Infections Related to Antibiotics** 103
José Ruiz Pardo and Clara Eugenia Cobo Cervantes

Editors' Contact Information 115

Index 117

Preface

Nosocomial infections are frequent complications after any type of surgery. Assuming that surgical site infection is the most frequent nosocomial infection, abdominal procedures imply the highest rates of all types of surgeries, as most elective abdominal techniques are clean-contaminated surgeries. The gastrointestinal and the genitourinary tracts have plenty of microorganisms, so once these cavities are entered, there is a potential extravasation of intraluminal content and consequently microorganisms. Furthermore, if we consider emergency procedures, we include contaminated and dirty techniques with exponentially higher bacterial contamination on the surgical field. When the contamination overcomes the chances of the immune system to control it, the nosocomial infection appears.

Nosocomial infections are associated with morbidity and mortality and reduce the patients´ quality of life after surgery. They also imply prolonged hospital stays and altogether they represent an economic burden for the Health Services.

Different guidelines have been published, describing recommendations for the prevention and treatment of nosocomial infections. These guidelines include pre, intra and postoperative measures, and refer not only to actions on the wound or the surgical field preparation, but also include systemic measures, such as prevention of hypothermia, control of hyperglycemia or reduction of tissue edema. Directed to specific nosocomial infection, like urinary or respiratory infection, these measures include avoidance of routine insertion of urinary catheter or postoperative early mobilization and respiratory physiotherapy. However, despite all these measures, nosocomial infections still represent a challenge for health-care staff. New measures are continuously appearing, trying to reduce the nosocomial infections rate. Along the same lines, new antibiotic weapons are arising to improve the control of the infection once it is present.

The aim of this book is to update the actual evidence on the different aspects of nosocomial infection after abdominal surgery, analyzing the diverse prophylactic measures and therapeutic weapons of the different types of nosocomial infections, but also revising the pathogenesis of these infections, the microrganisms involved and the perspectives of future for this life-threatening condition.

We hope that this book, based on the current evidence, can be helpful in the clinical practice. However, we must always keep in mind that medical investigation obtains new data, drugs and approaches every day, so that current evidence can be outdated in the following decade, requiring further updates.

Finally, we want to thank to all the contributing authors their availability, time and efforts to write all the chapters.

Jaime Ruiz-Tovar, MD, PhD
Andres Garcia-Marin, MD, PhD
Editors

Chapter 1

Epidemiology of Nosocomial Infection

José Ruiz Pardo[1],[*]
and Clara Eugenia Cobo Cervantes[2]

[1]Department of General and Digestive Surgery,
Hospital Universitario Torrecárdenas, Almería, Spain
[2]Department of Orthopaedic Surgery and Traumatology,
Hospital Universitario Torrecárdenas,
Almería, Spain

Abstract

The chapter summarizes the recent evidence about the epidemiology of the nosocomial infection. Moreover, other aspects such as impact, etiology and epidemiological surveillance are analyzed.

Keywords: infection, nosocomial infection, incidence, impact, infection etiology, risk factors

Introduction

Nosocomial infection is the most preventable cause of serious adverse events in hospitalized patients. These infections cause incalculable effects on their lives, deteriorate the image of healthcare teams, hospitals and the healthcare

---

[*] Corresponding Author's E-mail: josrp@hotmail.es.

In: Nosocomial Infection in Abdominal Surgery
Editors: Jaime Ruiz-Tovar and Andrés García Marín
ISBN: 978-1-68507-603-0
© 2022 Nova Science Publishers, Inc.

system, causing a huge impact on the country's economy and putting the sustainability of the healthcare system at risk [1].

Nosocomial infections are those acquired during the hospital stay and that were not present either in the incubation period or at the time of admission of the patient. Infections that occur more than 48 - 72 hours after admission are usually considered nosocomial infections [1, 2]. However, today the concept of healthcare-related infection has clearly transcended the hospital setting. Technological advances, which have facilitated the prolongation of life to very advanced ages, have led healthcare to non-strictly hospital settings. In this way, patients go to day centers for the control of their diseases, diagnostic techniques and surgical interventions of major surgery are practiced on an outpatient basis, ambulatory hemodialysis is performed, intravenous treatments are carried out at home, or they are admitted to social health centers for chronic or convalescent patients in whom health care of a certain complexity is provided [1].

In 2002, Friedman et al. [3] described that in patients not hospitalized but in contact with the healthcare system who presented bacteremia, this had foci and an etiology very similar to that of patients admitted to hospital, in contrast to those acquired in the community by patients strictly without contact with the healthcare system. For this reason, Friedman coined the term "healthcare-related infections" and proposed inclusion criteria that are currently in force:

Patient with positive blood cultures obtained during the first 48 hours after admission and any of the following criteria:

- Hospitalization at home with intravenous treatment.
- Specialized wound care in an outpatient center.
- Outpatient hemodialysis.
- Treatment with chemotherapy in the 30 days prior to bacteremia.
- Admission to an acute hospital for 2 or more days in the 90 days prior to bacteremia.
- Residence in a geriatric or long-term-stay center.

These criteria, which were well established for bacteremia, now they are applied to any healthcare-related infection in outpatients.

Frequency of Occurrence

About 5% of hospitalized patients develop a nosocomial infection during admission [1].

Regarding the order of frequency of nosocomial infections, respiratory tract infection accounted for 24%, surgical site infection 19%, urinary tract infection 17% and bacteremia associated with a vascular catheter 14% [4].

In the Intensive Care Units (ICU), the frequency of nosocomial infection in 2012 was 10.2%, where pneumonia accounted for 33.5%, urinary infection 30.5% and bacteremia 19% [2].

On the other hand, Clostridium difficile is the main cause of infectious nosocomial diarrhea in developed countries. In Europe, 80% of cases of C. *difficile* infection are acquired in hospitalized patients, 14% in the community and 6% are of indeterminate origin. The mean incidence of nosocomial cases is 4.1 cases per 10000 patient-days [5].

Impact of Nosocomial Infection

Nosocomial infections cause high mortality, prolong hospital stay and increase healthcare costs (1). According to data estimated by the National Nosocomial Infection Surveillance System (NNIS), during 2002 there were more than 1,7 million nosocomial infections and around 100000 deaths annually from this cause in the United States. For this reason, healthcare-related infections were among the 10 most common causes of death in that country [6].

The eradication of nosocomial infections is a utopia, since an inherent risk in any invasive procedure performed during hospitalization is unavoidable. However, the maximum reduction in the number of infections is possible through adequate prevention [1]. It has been estimated that the application of nosocomial infection prevention programs can prevent around 65% of bacteremia and urinary tract infections, as well as 55% of pneumonia and surgical infections, saving thousands of lives and millions of euros [7].

Etiology

Nosocomial infection is related to invasive care procedures, for example: catheter-associated bacteremia with vascular catheterization, urinary infection with urinary catheterization, respiratory infection with invasive mechanical ventilation and surgical infection with surgery [1].

All of them have in common the disruption of the host's own defenses by a device or an incision, allowing the invasion by microorganisms that are part of the patient's usual flora (endogenous flora), flora selected by selective antibiotic pressure (endogenous secondary flora), or flora found in the inanimate hospital setting (exogenous flora) [1].

The relative frequency of the different microorganisms varies depending on the focus. For example, staphylococcus aureus is the most frequent cause of pneumonia associated with mechanical ventilation and surgical infection, while escherichia coli is the most frequent cause of urinary tract infections and negative coagulase staphylococcus for catheter-associated bacteremia [1].

In ICUs, the most common microorganism isolated in nosocomial infections is pseudomonas aeruginosa (14.5%), followed by escherihia coli (13.5%), enterococcus faecalis (7.9%), klebsiella pneumoniae (7.5%), staphylococcus epidermidis (5.9%), candida albicans (5.1%), staphylococcus aureus (4.9%), acinetobacter baumanii (3.7%) and negative coagulase staphylococci (2.4%) [2].

Epidemiological Surveillance

Epidemiological surveillance is a vitally important instrument to identify, measure and analyze the health problem posed by nosocomial infection. Thus, it has formed the basis of infection control programs.

The main reasons for establishing epidemiological surveillance programs for nosocomial infection are: establish baseline infection rates, reduce the incidence of hospital infections, establish the efficacy of prevention measures, establish comparisons with other hospitals, detect outbreaks (grouping of cases in time and space), convince clinicians and managers of certain problems, and have defense measures against lawsuits.

Conclusion

About 5% of hospitalized patients develop a nosocomial infection during admission. Regarding the order of frequency of nosocomial infections, respiratory tract infection accounted for 24%, surgical site infection 19%, urinary tract infection 17% and bacteremia associated with a vascular catheter 14%.

In the Intensive Care Units (ICU), the frequency of nosocomial infection in 2012 was 10,2%, where pneumonia accounted for 33,5%, urinary infection 30,5% and bacteremia 19%. Clostridium difficile is the main cause of infectious nosocomial diarrhea in developed countries, with a mean incidence of 4,1 cases per 10000 patient-days.

Nosocomial infection is related to invasive care procedures: catheter-associated bacteremia with vascular catheterization, urinary infection with urinary catheterization, respiratory infection with invasive mechanical ventilation and surgical infection with surgery [1].

References

[1] Pujol, M., Limón, E. General epidemiology of nosocomial infections. Surveillance systems and programs. *Enferm Infecc. Microbiol. Clin.,* 2013; 31:108 - 13. Spanish.
[2] Zaragoza, R., Ramírez, P., López-Pueyo, M. J. Infección nosocomial en las unidades de cuidados intensivos [Nosocomial infections in intensive care units]. *Enferm Infecc. Microbiol. Clin.,* 2014; 32:320 - 7. Spanish.
[3] Friedman, N. D., Kaye, K. S., Stout, J. E., McGarry, S. A., Trivette, S. L., Briggs, J. P. et al. Health care-associated bloodstream infections in adults: A reason to change the accepted definition of community-acquired infections. *Ann. Intern. Med.,* 2002; 19:791 - 7.
[4] Zarb, P., Coignard, B., Griskeviciene, J., Muller, A., Vankerckhoven, V., Weist, K. et al. The European Centre for Disease Prevention and Control (ECDC) pilot point prevalence survey of healthcare-associated infections and antimicrobial use. *Euro Surveill.,* 2012; 17, pii: 20316.
[5] Bouza, E. Consequences of Clostridium difficile infection: Understanding the healthcare burden. *Clin. Microbiol. Infect.,* 2012 Dec.; 18 Suppl. 6:5 - 12.
[6] Klevens, R. M., Edwards, J. R., Richards, Jr. C. L., Horan, T. C., Gaynes, R. P., Pollock, D. A. et al. Estimating health care-associated infections and deaths in U.S. hospitals, 2002. *Public Health Rep.,* 2007; 122:160 - 6.
[7] Umscheid, C. A., Mitchell, M. D., Doshi, J. A., Agarwal, R., Williams, K., Brennan, P. J. Estimating the proportion of healthcare-associated infections that are reasonably preventable and the related mortality and costs. *Infect. Control Hosp. Epidemiol.,* 2011; 32:101 - 14.

Chapter 2

Risk Factors for Nosocomial Infection

Francisco Javier Ruescas García[1] and Celia Pérez Parra[2,*]

[1]Department of General and Digestive Surgery,
Hospital de Hellín, Albacete, Spain
[2]Department of Obstetrics and Gynecology,
Hospital de Almansa, Spain

Abstract

Patients with abdominal surgery are especially vulnerable to nosocomial infections due to various reasons, such as the disruption of many natural epithelial barriers, the immunosuppression associated with a surgical patient, orotracheal intubation in general anesthesia and the use of catheters and drains. Among the factors that increase the risk of nosocomial infection of the patient are extreme age, malnutrition, diabetes mellitus, previous radiation of the surgical site, hypothermia, hypoxemia, a coexisting infection distant from the surgical site, recent operation, swelling and hypocholesterolemia. We must implement nosocomial infection prevention programs as it has been shown that they can considerably reduce this type of infection.

Keywords: nosocomial infections, risk factors, abdominal surgery

---

[*] Corresponding Author's E-mail: ruescas4@hotmail.com.

In: Nosocomial Infection in Abdominal Surgery
Editors: Jaime Ruiz-Tovar and Andrés García Marín
ISBN: 978-1-68507-603-0
© 2022 Nova Science Publishers, Inc.

Introduction

Nosocomial infections are those contracted by a patient during his treatment in a hospital or another health center and whom patient did not have or was not incubating at the time of admission. Abdominal surgery patients are especially vulnerable to nosocomial infections directly related to the surgical procedure, such as surgical site infection or intra-abdominal infections, and to infections routinely related to invasive procedures, such as central venous access devices associated to bloodstream infections, urinary tract infections associated with catheters and pneumonia associated with mechanical ventilation, among others.

Pathogenesis

There are numerous reasons why the surgical patient is susceptible to nosocomial infections, including:

- The disruption of the natural epithelial barriers, allowing the invasion by microorganisms that are part of the patient's usual flora (endogenous flora), flora selected by selective antibiotic pressure (secondarily endogenous flora), or flora found in the inanimate hospital environment (exogenous flora)
- The immunosuppressive effect of surgical disease. During the surgical act, we cause trauma and burns that facilitate infection. Immunosuppression can also be due to drugs such as immunosuppressive treatment after transplantation of a solid organ or to frequent corticoid treatment in this type of patients. Patients with malignant tumor disease present an alteration of the immune system that also brings on nosocomial infection.
- General anesthesia, which generally involves orotracheal intubation, with mechanical ventilation and reduced consciousness time, increases the risk of pulmonary aspiration of gastric contents, with the consequent increased risk of pneumonia.

Classification

There are numerous risk factors described for nosocomial infection in patients with abdominal surgery, and more specifically for organ infections, such as surgical site infection, nosocomial pneumonia, urinary tract infection, and infection associated with intravascular catheterization. Risk factors can be classified into:

Risk Factors Linked to the Patient

Age
Advanced age is a well-known risk factor for nosocomial infections, producing immune aging. Damaged T cell function represents the most consistent and dramatic change. As early as in 1980s, Saviteer et al., described daily infection rates of 0.59 percent in patients older than 60 years and 0.40 percent in younger patients (relative risk: 1.49), with a daily incidence of urinary tract infections, respiratory infections and septicemia that increased significantly in elderly patients with risk ratios of 2.78, 2.07 and 1.36, respectively.

Malnutrition
The reestablishment of anabolism in acute critical illness requires calories and nitrogen more than basal requirements, of at least 25 kCal/kg/day. Inasmuch as, a large part of critically ill patients suffers from anorexia and in many times difficulty for oral intake, the macronutrient deficiency had been associated with an increase in nosocomial infections and other complications. Therefor, the benefit of early parenteral nutrition was postulated, but none of the trials showed a real benefit with this practice. In fact, Casaer et al., in a randomized, multicenter study with 4640 patients concluded that late initiation of parenteral nutrition was associated with faster recovery and fewer complications, compared to early initiation.

However, early enteral nutrition (< 48h), if there is no contraindication, has shown a significantly lower incidence of infections (relative risk reduction, 0.45; 95% confidence interval, 0.30-0.66; p .00006) and a reduction in hospital stay (mean reduction of 2.2 days; 95% confidence interval, 0.81-3.63 days; p .004) in seriously ill and injured patients according to a meta-analysis carried out by Marik and Zaloga.

Obesity

Obesity negatively affects immune function and host defense, characterized by a state of low-grade, chronic inflammation in addition to disturbed levels of circulating nutrients and metabolic hormones. Obesity is a significant risk factor for clinically relevant nosocomial infections in surgical patients as already demonstrated by Chovan at all, where they obtained rates of 0.05 percent in normal weight in a retrospective study, compared to 2.8 percent and 4.0 percent in the obese and severely obese groups ($P < 0.01$), wound infections being more frequent, followed by C. difficile infections, pneumonia, and bacteremia.

Later Cantürk et al., observed a significant increase in the total number of nosocomial infections in obese patients compared to normal weight patients ($p < 0.05$), describing high-density lipoprotein-cholesterol below the 10th percentile as a factor of independent risk for infection at the surgical site.

Diabetes Mellitus

Diabetic patients undergoing major abdominal surgery have an increased risk of infection and mortality that is further exacerbated by early postoperative hyperglycemia. Hyperglycemia induces immune cell dysfunction even if it is transient. It also increases catabolism and insulin resistance associated with surgical stress. Pomposelli el al described an infection risk rate of 2.7 times higher in patients with hyperglycemia > 220 mg/dL than in diabetic patients with glycemic levels less than < 220 mg/dL on the first postoperative day, increasing to the 5th, 7 the risk of infection if mild urinary infections are excluded. The first clinical trials that investigated the role of strictly controlled glucose levels (blood glucose < 110mg/dl) showed a marked benefit in the survival of critically ill patients, with a decrease in the rate of nosocomial infections, and organ dysfunction in postoperative patients. However, in a large international and randomized trial, NICE-SUGAR, found that intensive glucose control increased mortality among adults in the ICU, given a substantially increased risk of hypoglycemia.

- Other risk factors described for nosocomial infection in patients with abdominal surgery are prior radiation of the site, coexisting infection distant from the surgical site, corticosteroids treatment, recent operation (especially chest and abdomen), chronic inflammation, hypocholesterolemia, and swallowing disorders.

- The pathologies related to colonization by Staphylococcus aureus, frequent in patients with chronic kidney failure, liver cirrhosis or diabetes mellitus, also increase the risk of nosocomial infection, assuming a high risk of infection caused by this microorganism during hospital admission.

Risk Factors Linked to Treatment

Blood Transfusion
Transfusions are the cause of immunosuppression and an independent risk factor for the appearance of postoperative infection as described by Xiao el al in postoperative gastric cancer patients. Claridge et al., found a significantly higher infection rate ($P < 0.0001$) in transfused patients of 33.0% versus 7.6% in non-transfused patients in trauma patients. This risk of infection presented a clear exponential relationship, in patients who received between 0 and 15 transfusions ($R2$ to 0.757), being almost constant when the 15 units were exceeded. In a meta-analysis published by Hill et al., they have estimated a risk of postoperative bacterial infection of 3.45 (range, 1.43-15.15), with a p value < or 0.05. Therefore, it is essential to have a conservative attitude and transfuse only when necessary.

Hypothermia
Surgical patients under general anesthesia are especially at risk of developing hypothermia, due to exposure, infusion of a large volume of unheated fluids or blood products, or loss by evaporation during surgery. Hypothermia exerts multiple effects at the cellular level, impairing innate immune function and has been directly related to the development of sequelae such as coagulopathy, infection, acute myocardial events, and death after surgery.

Hypoxemia
Hypoxemia is due to injury to the airways, lungs, or chest wall, inability to maintain the airway, massive blood loss, cardiovascular instability, microcirculation alteration, or acute respiratory distress syndrome (ARDS). Patients with low partial pressure of tissue oxygen are more susceptible to wound infection and intestinal anastomotic leaks after colorectal surgery. It is also associated with peri-operative complications such as acute postoperative kidney injury, septic shock, and acute systemic inflammatory pathologies.

Inadequate Resuscitation Technique

The amount and type of fluids needed to reestablish hemodynamics and tissue perfusion is still under discussion. Delaney et al., in a meta-analysis that included 17 studies concluded that the use of solutions containing albumin for resuscitation of patients with sepsis was associated with lower mortality compared to other fluid resuscitation regimens.

- Other notable risk factors linked to treatment are emergency surgery procedures, excessive use of drains, inadequate antibiotic prophylaxis, prolonged surgical time and prolonged preoperative hospitalization.

Environmental Risk Factors

- Environmental risk factors for nosocomial infection have been extensively studied in trials dedicated to the study of surgical site infection. These include inadequate disinfection, poor skin antisepsis, inadequate ventilation, and contaminated medication. These factors are potentially preventable and have been included in the checklists and packages of measures, the applicability of which has led to a reduction in the number of nosocomial infections, as discussed below.

Prevention

Nosocomial infection can be prevented to a certain extent, and all necessary measures must be taken to do so.

First, we must perform a complete preoperative evaluation to identify and quantify any concomitant pathology that may influence a negative surgical result. We can use tools to adjust risk and improve postoperative results, creating predictive models of morbidity and mortality, such as the National Surgical Quality Improvement Program. Within these measures, a complete evaluation of the functional and cognitive status of the patient is essential, ruling out the presence of cognitive impairment or dementia, depression, alcohol or other substance abuse, cardiac risk factors, lung, kidney and hepatobiliary function, nutritional status, endocrine disorders such as Diabetes

Mellitus and medication management. Any of these alterations should be corrected or optimized preoperatively to improve the postoperative prognosis.

Parenteral antibiotic prophylaxis should be administered in the hour prior to the surgical incision, with intraoperative re-dosing if necessary due to prolonged surgical time or bleeding, not exceeding 24 hours of prophylaxis (preferably single dose). Prolonged prophylaxis increases the risk of nosocomial infections not related to the surgical site and the risk of multi-resistant pathogens. For surgical preparation of the skin prior to surgical incision, chlorhexidine used as skin antiseptic at concentrations of 0.5 to 4% has bactericidal, virucidal and fungicidal action and has been shown to be superior to povidone-iodine solution for infection of the surgical site.

During the hospital stay, it must be considered that hand washing is the most effective method to reduce the spread of pathogen transmission. Regarding catheters and drains, we must avoid their use if they are not necessary and remove them as soon as possible. For its insertion, the appropriate type of drainage must be chosen, the skin adequately prepared, protective barrier measures applied, and the appropriate dressing applied. We must maintain the same hygiene measures for wound healing and dressing changes. The universal precautionary measures (gloves, mask, cap, gown, and eye protection) should be used in case of risk of splashing body fluids.

According to Umscheid et al., the application of nosocomial infection prevention programs can prevent around 65-70% of bacteremia and urinary tract infections and 55% of pneumonia and surgical infections. In the Spanish Health System, a series of projects are being developed to reduce the rate of nosocomial infection, such as the Zero Surgical Infection Project, Zero Bacteremia and Zero pneumonia.

Conclusion

Abdominal surgery patients are especially vulnerable to nosocomial infections, with numerous risk factors involved for such infections. Given that part of these risk factors is modifiable to reduce nosocomial infections, we must take the necessary measures to prevent them, being of the utmost importance the application of nosocomial infection prevention programs.

References

Abdelmalak B B, Cata J P, Bonilla A, You J, Kopyeva T, Vogel J D, Campbell S, Sessler D I. Intraoperative tissue oxygenation and postoperative outcomes after major non-cardiac surgery: an observational study. *Br. J. Anaesth.* 2013;110(2):241-9. doi: 10.1093/ bja/aes378. Epub 2012 Nov 21. PMID: 23171726.

Barie S, Philip. "Surgical infections and Antibiotic Use." In *Sabinston* T*extbox of Surgery: The Biológical Basics of Modern Surgical Practice.* Edited by Coutney M. Townsend, Jr, 241-280. Philadelphia: Elsevier, 2017. ISBN978-0-323-40162-7.

Cantürk Z, Cantürk N Z, Cetinarslan B, Utkan N Z, Tarkun I. Nosocomial infections and obesity in surgical patients. *Obes. Res.* 2003;11(6):769-75. doi: 10.1038/oby.2003.107. PMID: 12805398.

Casaer M P, Mesotten D, Hermans G, Wouters P J, Schetz M, Meyfroidt G, Van Cromphaut S, Ingels C, Meersseman P, Muller J, Vlasselaers D, Debaveye Y, Desmet L, Dubois J, Van Assche A, Vanderheyden S, Wilmer A, Van den Berghe G. Early versus late parenteral nutrition in critically ill adults. *N. Engl. J. Med.* 2011 Aug 11;365(6):506-17. doi: 10.1056/NEJMoa1102662. Epub 2011 Jun 29. PMID: 21714640.

Cheadle W G. Risk factors for surgical site infection. *Surg. Infect. (Larchmt).* 2006;7 Suppl 1:S7-11. doi: 10.1089/sur.2006.7.s1-7. PMID: 16834549.

Choban P S, Heckler R, Burge J C, Flancbaum L. Increased incidence of nosocomial infections in obese surgical patients. *Am. Surg.* 1995 Nov;61(11):1001-5. PMID: 7486411.

Claridge J A, Sawyer R G, Schulman A M, McLemore E C, Young J S. Blood transfusions correlate with infections in trauma patients in a dose-dependent manner. *Am. Surg.* 2002;68(7):566-72. PMID: 12132734.

Darouiche R O, Wall M J Jr, Itani K M, Otterson M F, Webb A L, Carrick M M, Miller H J, Awad S S, Crosby C T, Mosier M C, Alsharif A, Berger D H. Chlorhexidine-Alcohol versus Povidone-Iodine for Surgical-Site Antisepsis. *N. Engl. J. Med.* 2010 Jan 7;362(1):18-26. doi: 10.1056/NEJMoa0810988. PMID: 20054046.

Delaney A P, Dan A, McCaffrey J, Finfer S. The role of albumin as a resuscitation fluid for patients with sepsis: a systematic review and meta-analysis. *Crit. Care Med.* 2011 Feb;39(2):386-91. doi: 10.1097/ CCM.0b013e3181ffe217. PMID: 21248514.

Dickinson A, Qadan M, Polk H C Jr. Optimizing surgical care: a contemporary assessment of temperature, oxygen, and glucose. *Am. Surg.* 2010;76(6):571-7. PMID: 20583510.

Gardner E M, Murasko D M. Age-related changes in Type 1 and Type 2 cytokine production in humans. *Biogerontology*. 2002;3(5):271-90. doi: 10.1023/a: 1020151401826. PMID: 12237564.

Govinda, R, Kasuya Y, Bala E, Mahboobi R, Devarajan J, Sessler D I, Akça O. Early postoperative subcutaneous tissue oxygen predicts surgical site infection. *Anesth. Analg.* 2010;111(4):946-52. doi: 10.1213/ANE .0b013e3181e80a94. PMID: 20601453.

Griesdale D E, Russell J de Souza, Rob M van Dam, Daren K Heyland, Deborah J Cook, Atul Malhotra, Rupinder Dhaliwal, William R Henderson, Dean R Chittock, Simon Finfer and Daniel Talmor. Intensive insulin therapy and mortality among critically ill patients: a meta-analysis including NICE-SUGAR study data. *CMAJ*. 2009. 180: 821–827.

Hill G E, Frawley W H, Griffith K E, Forestner J E, Minei J P. Allogeneic blood transfusion increases the risk of postoperative bacterial infection: a meta-analysis. *J. Trauma.* 2003;54(5):908-14. doi: 10. 1097/01.TA.000 0022460.21283.53. PMID: 12777903.

Ingels C, Vanhorebeek I, Van den Berghe G. Glucose homeostasis, nutrition and infections during critical illness. *Clin. Microbiol. Infect.* 2018;24(1):10-15. doi: 10.1016/j.cmi.2016.12.033. Epub 2017 Jan 7. PMID: 28082192.

Ives C L, Harrison D K, Stansby G S. Tissue oxygen saturation, measured by near-infrared spectroscopy, and its relationship to surgical-site infections. *Br. J. Surg. 2007*;94(1):87-91. doi: 10.1002/bjs.5533. PMID: 17054313.

Marik P E, Zaloga G P. Early enteral nutrition in acutely ill patients: a systematic review. *Crit. Care Med.* 2001 Dec;29(12):2264-70. doi: 10. 1097/00003246-200112000-00005.

Milner J J, Beck M A. The impact of obesity on the immune response to infection. *Proc. Nutr. Soc.* 2012 May;71(2):298-306. doi: 10.1017/ S002966 5112000158. Epub 2012 Mar 14. PMID: 22414338; PMCID: PMC4791086.

Mueck K M, Kao L S. Patients at High-Risk for Surgical Site Infection. *Surg. Infect. (Larchmt).* 2017 May/Jun;18(4):440-446. doi: 10.1089/ sur.2017.058. Epub 2017 Apr 12. PMID: 28402740.

Namias N, Harvill S, Ball S, McKenney M G, Salomone J P, Civetta J M. Cost and morbidity associated with antibiotic prophylaxis in the ICU. *J. Am. Coll. Surg.* 1999 Mar;188(3):225-30. doi: 10.1016/s1072-7515(98)00287-7. PMID: 10065809.

NICE-SUGAR Study Investigators. Intensive versus conventional glucose control in critically ill patients. *N. Engl. J. Med.* 2009;360:1283-97.

Organización Panamericana de la Salud. Prevención y control de infecciones asociadas a la saud. *Recomendaciones Básicas*. Washington, D.C.: 2017. ISBN: 978-92-75-31954-3. [Prevention and control of infections associated with health. *Basic Recommendations*]

Pilmis, B, T Billard-Pomares, M Martin, D Seytre, E Carbonnelle and J-R Zahar. Can environmental contamination be explained by particular traits associated with patients?. *Journal of Hospital Infection*. 2020;104: 293 – 297.

Pomposelli J J, Baxter J K 3rd, Babineau T J, Pomfret E A, Driscoll D F, Forse R A, Bistrian B R. Early postoperative glucose control predicts nosocomial infection rate in diabetic patients. *JPEN J. Parenter Enteral Nutr*. 1998 Mar-Apr;22(2):77-81. doi: 10.1177/0148607 19802200277. PMID: 9527963.

Pronovost, Peter, Dale Needham, Sean Berenholtz, David Sinopoli, Haitao Chu, Sara Cosgrove, Bryan Sexton, Robert Hyzy, Robert Welsh, Gary Roth, Joseph Bander, John Kepros and Christine Goeschel. An intervention to decrease catheter-related bloodstream infections in the ICU. *N. Engl. J. Med*. 2006;355:2725–32.

Pujol M, Limón E. Epidemiología general de las infecciones nosocomiales. Sistemas y programas de vigilancia [General epidemiology of nosocomial infections. Surveillance systems and programs]. *Enferm. Infecc. Microbiol. Clin*. 2013 Feb;31(2):108-13. Spanish. doi: 10.1016/j.eimc.2013.01.001. Epub 2013 Jan 26. PMID: 23357654.

Qadan M, Gardner S A, Vitale D S, Lominadze D, Joshua I G, Polk H C Jr. Hypothermia and surgery: immunologic mechanisms for current practice. *Ann. Surg*. 2009 Jul;250(1):134-40. doi: 10.1097/SLA. 0b013e3181ad85f7. PMID: 19561472; PMCID: PMC2811072.

Qadan M, Weller E B, Gardner S A, Maldonado C, Fry D E, Polk H C Jr. Glucose and surgical sepsis: a study of underlying immunologic mechanisms. *J. Am. Coll. Surg*. 2010 Jun;210(6):966-74. doi: 10.1016/j.jamcollsurg.2010.02.001. Epub 2010 Apr 28. PMID: 20510806.

Reintam Blaser A, Starkopf J, Alhazzani W, Berger M M, Casaer M P, Deane A M, Fruhwald S, Hiesmayr M, Ichai C, Jakob S M, Loudet C I, Malbrain M L, Montejo González J C, Paugam-Burtz C, Poeze M, Preiser J C, Singer P, van Zanten A R, De Waele J, Wendon J, Wernerman J, Whitehouse T, Wilmer A, Oudemans-van Straaten H M; ESICM Working Group on Gastrointestinal Function. Early enteral nutrition in critically ill patients: ESICM clinical practice guidelines. *Intensive Care Med*. 2017 Mar;43(3):380-398. doi: 10.1007/s00134-016-4665-0. Epub 2017 Feb 6. PMID: 28168570; PMCID: PMC5323492.

Saviteer S M, Samsa G P, Rutala W A. Nosocomial infections in the elderly. Increased risk per hospital day. *Am. J. Med*. 1988;84(4):661-6. doi: 10.1016/0002-9343(88)90101-5. PMID: 3400661.

Umscheid C A, Mitchell M D, Doshi J A, Agarwal R, Williams K, Brennan P J. Estimating the proportion of healthcare-associated infections that are reasonably preventable and the related mortality and costs. *Infect. Control*

Hosp. Epidemiol. 2011 Feb; 32(2):101-14. doi: 10.1086/ 657912. PMID: 21460463.

Umscheid C A, Mitchell M D, Doshi J A, Agarwal R, Williams K, Brennan P J. Estimating the proportion of healthcare-associated infections that are reasonably preventable and the related mortality and costs. *Infect. Control Hosp. Epidemiol.* 2011 Feb;32(2):101-14. doi: 10.1086/ 657912. PMID: 21460463.

Xiao H, Quan H, Pan S, Yin B, Luo W, Huang G, Ouyang Y. Impact of peri-operative blood transfusion on post-operative infections after radical gastrectomy for gastric cancer: a propensity score matching analysis focusing on the timing, amount of transfusion and role of leukocyte depletion. *J. Cancer Res. Clin. Oncol.* 2018;144(6):1143-1154. doi: 10.1007/s00432-018-2630-8. Epub 2018 Mar 23. PMID: 29572591; PMCID: PMC5948291.

Chapter 3

Prophylactic Measures against Surgical Site Infection after Abdominal Surgery

Jaime Ruiz-Tovar[*], MD, PhD
Department of Surgery, Universidad Rey Juan Carlos, Madrid, Spain

Abstract

In the last years, diverse scientific societies have published different guidelines including recommendations to reduce the risk of developing a postoperative surgical site infections. These measures can be applied pre- intra and postoperatively and joined in a bundle, they might have a synergistic effect on the prevention of the infections.

The aim of the present chapter is to summarize the most relevant measures for surgical site infection prevention.

Keywords: surgical site infections, prophylaxis, abdominal surgery

Introduction

Surgical site infection (SSI) is defined as an infection that occurs within 30 days after surgery in the part of the body where a previous surgical act took place. Depending on the depth of affection, SSI may be superficial incisional

---

[*] Corresponding Author's E-mail: jruiztovar@gmail.com.

In: Nosocomial Infection in Abdominal Surgery
Editors: Jaime Ruiz-Tovar and Andrés García Marín
ISBN: 978-1-68507-603-0
© 2022 Nova Science Publishers, Inc.

infections (involving the skin only) or deep incisional infections, or infections involving organs or cavities, defined as organ-space SSI.

SSIs are the most frequently reported nosocomial infections, accounting for 30% of such infections among hospitalized patients. Moreover, SSI is implicated in one-third of postoperative deaths and accounts for 8% of all deaths caused by a nosocomial infection. Furthermore, SSI incurs considerable increases in healthcare costs. However, the incidence of SSI widely varies between procedures, hospitals, surgeons and patients.

In most SSIs, the responsible pathogens originate from the patient's endogenous flora. The most commonly microorganisms involved in the development of SSI are grampositive cocci, gramnegative bateriae and anaerobic agents. According to the degree of contamination, surgeries can be classified as clean, clean-contaminated, contaminated or dirty procedures. The most commonly isolated organisms in clean surgery are *Staphylococcus aureus* and coagulase negative staphylococci, whereas in clean-contaminated or contaminated surgery; the most frequent organisms are *Enterococcus* spp. and *Escherichia coli*.

As SSIs are still a challenge for surgeons, representing a health burden for the sanitary systems, many researches are focused on developing measures to reduce the incidence of this complication. In the last years, diverse scientific societies have developed protocols or recommendation documents including several measures to decrease the risk of SSI. Among this organizations we can include the World Health Organization (WHO), the Center for Disease Control (CDC), the Surgical Infection Society (SIS) or the American College of Surgeons (ACS) [1-3].

Three factors are considered the determinants for SSI: the surgeon, the patient and the microorganism. The patient is the factor with less ability for modification. However, the patient can be optimized before surgery. The most relevant factors related to the patient amenable for optimization are the improvement of the nutritional status, the reduction of obesity, the optimization of comorbidities and the cessation of the tobacco habit [1].

Referring to the pattern of microorganisms causing infection, it has been observed that they have not significantly changed during the last decades. However, the rate of bacteria resistant to antibiotics has increased. This is the result of a bad politics of antibiotic administration with excessive, inadequate, and prolonged prescriptions. Diverse programs have been developed to optimize the use of antibiotics, aiming to reduce the prevalence of multiresistant bacteria, that finally lead to increased rates of SSIs and in a more severe manner [1-3].

Finally, the surgeon is considered the main modulator of SSI. Surgical experience and skills have shown to reduce the incidence of SSIs. A correct tissular management, adequate hemostasia, reduction of extravasation of intraluminal content, among others are surgical maneuvers associated with reduced complications risk. Furthermore, the surgeon has pharmacologic and non-pharmacologic measures to reduce bacterial contamination and, consequently, the incidence of SSI [1]. The most relevant recommendations will be discussed here.

Adequate Nutritional Support

Nowadays the relationship between nutritional status and the immune system is well known. Desnutrition impairs immune response may make patients highly susceptible to postoperative infections, hence patients with desnutrition may suffer a range of poor outcomes including increased risk of death, sepsis and poor wound healing [4, 5].

Nutrition preoperative support intervention in patients identified by screening and assessment as at risk for malnutrition or malnourished may improve clinical outcomes. Nutrition intervention in malnourished patients was associated with improved nutrition status, nutrient intake, physical function, and quality of life. In addition, hospital readmissions were reduced. Considering the high prevalence of malnutrition and its repercussions in patient morbidity-mortality and healthcare cost, nutritional screening measures must be included in an integrated nutritional care plan for patients while in the hospital. Perioperative nutritional screening (PONS) score has been specifically designed for use in perioperative period is the reason why we recommend implementing this screening tool in surgical patients [6, 7].

PONS Questions for Clinic-Based Perioperative Nutrition Screening

- Does the patient have a low BMI <18.5 kg/m2 (<20 in >65 y of age)?
- Has the patient experienced a weight loss >10% in past 6 months?
- Has the patient had a reduced oral intake by >50% in the past week? (and/or)
- Does the patient have a preoperative serum albumin <3.0 g/dL?

According to the PONS score subdivide patient in two categories:

Nutrition Pathway in Low Nutrition Risk Perioperative Patients

(i.e., PONS <1 and Albumin [ALB] >3.0).

Patients should be encouraged to take in healthy high-protein (with high-quality protein sources, such as eggs, fish, and lean meats/dairy) complex carbohydrate-rich diets preoperatively. However, many patients will not be able to meet optimal suggested perioperative energy goals of 25 kcal/kg/d and 1.5–2 g/kg/d of protein from routine food intake. Thus, patients are encouraged to take high-protein ONSs (oral nutritional supplements) or IMN (immunonutrition) during the perioperative period unrelated to nutritional status [7].

Nutrition Pathway in Patients found to be at Nutrition Risk

(i.e., PONS >1 or ALB <3.0).

In patients found to be at nutrition risk, high-protein ONS or IMN are recommended preoperatively. This should have a goal of delivering at least 1.2 g/kg/d total of protein. High-protein ONS should contain >18 g/protein/serving in a balanced formula. A reasonable goal for most patients is 3 high-protein ONS servings per day. Previous data utilizing preoperative ONS demonstrated benefits on reduction of surgical-site infections in selected weight-losing patients. As many patients do not meet their energy needs from regular food, especially malnourished patients, it is encouraged the use of high-protein ONS or IMN [8, 9].

In this context, there are some meta-analyses showing that a multiple nutrient-enhanced nutritional formula (arginine, glutamine, omega 3, fatty acids, nucleotides) was associated with significantly reduced SSI incidence compared with a standard formula. WHO recommends that multiple nutrient enhanced formulas can be used to prevent SSIs in adult patients undergoing major surgery, nevertheless some factors could be considered such as resources and product availability should be carefully assessed, particularly in settings with limited resources [10].

It is recommended that patients at nutritional risk before major surgery receive preoperative ONSs for a period of at least 7 days. This may be achieved with either IMN formulas or high-protein ONS. When oral nutrition supplementation via ONS is not possible, indication for enteral nutrition for a period of at least 7 days must be evaluated. If neither oral nutrition supplementation via ONS nor enteral nutrition are possible preoperative parenteral nutrition may be indicated to improve outcomes.

In normal conditions preoperative fasting from midnight must be abandoned. Patients undergoing surgery who are considered to have minimal specific risk of aspiration, we encourage unrestricted access to solids for up to 8 h before anesthesia and clear fluids for oral intake up to 2 h before the induction of anesthesia. It is recommended a preoperative carbohydrate drink containing at least 45 g of carbohydrate to improve insulin sensitivity (except in type I diabetics due to their insulin deficiency state). Complex carbohydrate (e.g., maltodextrin) should be used when available [11].

Postoperative Nutritional Intervention

Postoperative nutritional support is vital in maintaining nutritional status during the catabolic postoperative period and underscored by evidence for early and sustained feeding after surgery [12].

A high-protein diet (via diet or high-protein ONS) must be initiated on the day of surgery in most cases, with exception of patients without bowel in continuity, with bowel ischemia, or persistent bowel obstruction. Traditional "clear liquid" and "full liquid" diets should not be routinely used. An overall protein intake goal is more important than total calorie intake in the postoperative period.

In patients started on nutritional intervention (oral supplementation, or enteral or parenteral nutrition), it is recommended to maintain it in the postoperative course until the patients can take at least 60% of their protein/kcal requirements via regular diet. After hospital discharge, the maintenance of high-protein ONS is recommended after major surgery, to meet both calorie and protein needs, especially in the previously malnourished, elderly and sarcopenic patient [12].

Preoperative Bath

Whole body bathing or showering with soap or skin antiseptics is a widespread practice before surgery to reduce skin resident and transient bacteria. However the most important question is whether preoperative bathing or showering with antiseptics reduce the incidence of SSI in comparison with their potential for harm such as changes in patterns of bacteria resistance, skin hipersensitivity, etc.

Webster and Osborne reviewed randomized clinical trials comparing antiseptic preparation (4% chlorhexidine gluconate) for preoperative bathing or showering with non-antiseptic preparations or no washing over a 26-year period between 1983 and 2009 (seven trials with 10.157 participants). The authors concluded that there was no clear evidence of benefit for preoperative showering or bathing with chlorhexidine over other wash products to reduce SSI [13].

Chlebicki et al. performed a meta-analysis of sixteen trials involving 17.932 patients, 7.952 received a chlorhexidine bath and 9.980 with others. Chlorhexidine bathing did not significantly reduce overal incidence of SSI when compared with soap, placebo or no shower or bath [14].

Preoperative Shave

Preparation the patient for surgery has traditionally included the routine hair removal from the incision site because its presence can interfere with the exposure, the suturing and the application of adhesive drapes. However some studies claim that preoperative hair removal is harmful, increase SSI and should be avoided [15, 16].

Hair can be removed by several different ways which include shaving, clipping the hair and using a chemical creams. Shaving is the commonest and cheapest method. During the process of shaving, the skin may experience microscopic cuts and abrasions. It is believed that microorganisms are able to colonize these cuts, thus contaminating the surgical incision site and causing wound infections. Thus, clippers are thought to reduce the risk of cuts and abrasions because do not come into contact with the patient's skin. This hair removal practice can be done everywhere (home, wards, theaters...) but research has suggested, that hair removal should not take place in the operating theatre as loose hair may contaminate the sterile surgical field [17].

Several trials that compared shaving with clipping showed significantly more SSI associated with shaving. Tanner et al. concluded in their meta-analysis that there was no significantly differences between hair removal and not hair removal; however, when it is necessary to remove hair, the evidence suggests that clippers are associated with fewer SSI than razors [15].

Antibiotic Prophylaxis

Indications for antibiotic prophylaxis depend on the type of surgery. Antibiotic prophylaxis is not always needed for clean surgery since the rate of SSI is very low; it should only be administered in some patients such as oncological and plastic breast surgery, intravascular devices placement, splenectomy in immunosuppression situations and mesh placement in high risk patients [18-20]. Antibiotic prophylaxis is always needed in clean-contaminated and contaminated procedures; however, it is still unclear in elective laparoscopic cholecystectomy in low-risk patients, considering as high risk patients those ones under immunosuppressive therapy or disease, ASA $\geq$III, acute or chronic cholecystitis 6 weeks before surgery, conversion to open surgery or intraoperative rupture of the gallbladder [21].

General principles of antibiotic prophylaxis are intravenous administration and selection of adequate antibiotic with correct posology. The antibiotic should present a narrow spectrum to cover the typical microorganisms, bactericidal actitiy, extended half life, good tissue distribution and low adverse effects. According to this, the recommended antibiotic for digestive surgeries above the duodenum, neck and breast surgeries would be cefazolin and, in patients with β-lactam allergies, vancomycin and gentamicin, clindamycin and gentamicin or levofloxacin. For digestive surgeries below the duodenum, amoxicillin-clavulanic and, in patients with β-lactam allergies, moxifloxacin, levofloxacin and metronidazole or gentamicin and metronidazole are preferred. The administration should be performed 30-60 minutes before the start of the procedure [2, 22].

Intraoperative redosing is recommended when there is a bleeding greater than 1500 ml or the surgical procedure lasts for more than two half-lifes of the antibiotic. Postoperative redosing in clean and clean-contaminated surgeries is not recommended with high level of evidence once the surgical incision has been closed, even if drainage is required [2, 22].

Dosing adjustment should be performed according to the patient comorbidities and weight, since the alteration in body composition in obese patients involves a higher risk of erroneous dosing and, therefore, a possible therapeutic failure or toxicity [23].

Surgical Skin Preparation

The goal of surgical site skin preparation with antiseptics is to reduce the microbial load of the skin before incision and, therefore, decreasing the incidence of SSI [1]. Decontamination of the skin is a standard of care that must always be carried out before any invasive procedure [24, 25].

The three agents mostly used in the surgical site skin preparation are chlorhexidine gluconate, povidone iodine and alcohols, although there are many more available options [24].

The alcoholic compounds are the most microbiologically active agents, but its anti-microbial effect disappears after a few minutes, are inflammable and contraindicated on mucosae membranes. Its use for surgical preparation has therefore been practically discontinued. Antiseptics such as chlorhexidine gluconate and povidone iodine are less active than alcohol but have a greater residual effect. Both can be found in aqueous or alcoholic solutions, the latter being more effective [16].

There are several randomized clinical trials that have compared chlorhexidine-based antiseptics with iodine-based antiseptics in the preoperative preparation of the skin. Most of them have been underpowered to detect differences in SSI rates [3]. The WHO recommendations concluded that alcohol-based antiseptics solutions were more effective than aqueous solutions in reducing the risk of SSI. More specifically, a decrease in SSI risk was observed when comparing the use of alcoholic chlorhexidine with aqueous povidone iodine [1]. However, it is important to bear in mind that these studies are comparing two antiseptics combined (chlorhexidine and alcohol) against just one (povidone iodine), but in combination present a greater reduction of SSI risk.

Adhesives Drapes

Adhesive plastic incise drapes are used on a patient's skin after surgical site preparation, with or without antimicrobial impregnation, and the surgeon performs the incision of the drape and the skin simultaneously. In available guidelines, there are conflicting recommendations on the use of plastic adhesive drapes, mainly discouraging their use. Results from non-randomized studies are controversial about the efficacy of this approach. A recent meta-analysis [26] assessed the impact of adhesive drapes on SSI comparing adhesive drapes versus no drape, and iodine-impregnated adhesive drapes versus no drape. SSI rates were higher in the adhesive drape groups; iodine impregnation was not associated with any significant difference in SSI. Another meta-analysis assessing adhesive drapes with and without antiseptic impregnation [27] found no benefit in terms of SSI. In addition, some allergic reactions occurred with impregnated drapes.

Considering this evidence, including availability and costs, actual recommendations do not support the use of adhesive incise drapes (with or without antimicrobial properties) for the purpose of preventing SSI.

Wound Protectors

The initial idea relied on the principle of reducing exposure of the surgical site to bacteria inherent in the surrounding skin or to airborne bacteria in the operating room. Major applicability was expected in clean surgeries, where the skin is considered the main source of bacteria. Several devices have been developed based on the concept of combining a non-traumatic surgical wound retractor with a protective membrane covering the incisional margin in abdominal surgeries. Wound protectors were hypothesized to reduce intraoperative contamination while concomitantly preserving the temperature and humidity of the surgical wound Diverse RCT demonstrated that wound protectors were efficacious in reducing the incidence of incisional SSI as compared to usual care in patients undergoing gastrointestinal surgeries. There are different circular wound edge protectors, consisting in devices with a single semirigid plastic ring placed into the abdominal cavity or devices with two semi-rigid plastic rings connected by an impervious drape [28].

Furthermore, the device is intended to facilitate the retraction of the incision during surgery without the need for additional mechanical retractors and cloths. Theoretically, commercially available wound protectors are intended to reduce wound edge contamination to a minimum during abdominal surgical procedures, including contamination from outside (clean surgery) and inside the peritoneal cavity (clean-contaminated, contaminated and dirty surgery) [29].

According to the actual evidence, it is recommended the use of CWEP devices in clean-contaminated, contaminated, and dirty abdominal surgical procedures for the purpose of reducing the rate of SSI.

Prophylactic Vacuum Therapy

Incisional negative pressure wound therapy (NPWT) has emerged as a useful tool to reduce surgical site infections [1]. Different devices have been developed to prevent complications via application immediately after surgery in high-risk closed surgical incisions. NPWT involves the controlled application of continuous sub-atmospheric pressure to the wound. While NPWT technology is an established and accepted treatment for non-healing wounds and open surgical incisions following infection, a growing number of clinical studies have been published based on the hypothesis that negative pressure dressings improve healing of closed wounds.

Surgical incisions disrupt the cutaneous layer that normally doesn't let bacteria entering the body. In healthy people it takes three to six days for reepithelialization to restore the barrier function of the skin. Risk factors such as diabetes or contaminated surgical fields such as related to abdominal surgical procedures with intestinal anastomoses result in prolonged time to healing. Post-operative colonization of surgical sites is associated with increased risk of SSI [30, 31].

Well-described mechanisms of action of incisional NPWT include protection of the incision site from external infectious sources and help in holding incision edges together [32]. Incisional NPWT also removes fluids and infectious materials from the surgical site, which is especially important in critical anatomical locations. Other mechanisms of action, particularly at the cellular and molecular level, are less understood and the subject of ongoing research [32, 33].

NPWT's ways to prevent SSIs includes eliminating dead space, removing fluid and blood, improving blood flow and preventing the formation of subcutaneous seromas/hematomas that become secondarily infected. In addition, NPWT is thought to decrease local inflammatory response and cell death by increasing the oxygen gradient across a wound.

The NPWT implies a continuous amount of sub-atmospheric pressure applied for several post-operative days. Most studies report use of -80 or -125mm Hg of sub-atmospheric pressure, for a length of five to seven days after operation.

NPWT seems to be effective in the prevention of SSI acting as a barrier which avoids bacteria contamination of the wound before healing, improving the lymphatic and blood flow, reducing seroma, hematoma, edema, and wound dehiscence [1]. This suggests that NPWT might be effective in reducing the risk of SSI in all types of surgical procedures. However, because of the elevated costs of the devices, diverse societies just recommend considering NPWT for high-risk surgical wounds [1].

Antimicrobial Sutures

The use of sutures coated or embedded with antiseptic are preventive measures against SSI, that can be implemented by the surgeon. Several studies have demonstrated that the suture used for the aponeurotic closure is a relevant factor that might influence the incidence of SSI. Bacteria adhere to the filaments of the suture, especially in multifilament ones. Thus, monofilament sutures are widely recommended for fascial closures, as with these sutures there is a lower place for bacterial accommodation.

In abdominal surgery, bacterial contamination comes from the digestive tract (*Enterobacteriaceae* and anaerobic microorganisms) and from the saprophytic flora of the skin (gram-positive). Sutures coated with antiseptic agents were designed to form a barrier against the bacterial transit from the intraperitoneal cavity to the subcutaneous tissue, that might lead to the development of incisional SSI. Moreover, their bactericide effect would prevent from bacterial adhesion to the suture filaments.

The most employed antiseptic agent used to coat the sutures is Triclosan (2,4,4-trichloro-2-hydroxi-diphenileter). In preclinical studies, Triclosan has demonstrated to reduce the bacterial load in the wound and to slow bacterial growth, inhibiting the synthesis of bacterial fatty acids.

Triclosan-coated sutures have been analyzed in different surgical procedures in humans, though most of them were conducted in clean and clean-contaminated ones. Among them, colorectal surgery has been the most widely procedure investigated, as the high incisional SSI rates that present, make these approaches as the most amenable to perform investigations on them. However, Triclosan-coated sutures have also demonstrated their efficacy in dirty surgery. A previous study of our group evaluated the efficacy of Triclosan-coated sutures in fecal peritonitis, revealing that the use of these sutures might reduce the incidence of incisional SSI in up to 80%.

Several meta-analyses have been published, evaluating the efficacy of Triclosan-coated sutures, demonstrating all of them a reduction in SSI rates, ranging from 24% to 84%. Furthermore, diverse organizations and societies have published recommendations, supporting the use of Triclosan-coated sutures. The WHO established a conditional recommendation, as coated sutures are more expensive, and their availability is limited in many countries.

However, the uses of Triclosan-coated sutures might reduce mean hospital stay and, consequently, sanitary costs [1].

The American College of Surgeons and the Surgical Infection Society support their use exclusively for the suture of aponeurotic layers, subcutaneous tissue, and skin in abdominal surgeries, but their use is not justified for visceral sutures. The contamination grade must be clean or clean-contaminated, but there is not enough evidence to justify their use in contaminated or dirty procedures [3].

Conclusion

The guidelines of the different scientific societies with recommendations to reduce the risk of SSIs are based on different studies demonstrating that the application of these measures are associated with a reduction of SSIs. The application of these measures individually might reduce the SSIs rate, but the combination of them within a bundle have demonstrated addition benefits. Actually, there is not an universally accepted bundle, but the greater the number of measures implemented, the greater the benefit. New measures are continuously arising, and therefore the guidelines must be periodically updated.

References

[1] Allegranzi B, Zayed B, Bischoff P, et al. New WHO recommendations on intraoperative and postoperative measures for surgical site infection prevention: an evidence-based global perspective. *Lancet Infect Dis.* 2016;16:e288-e303.

[2] Berríos-Torres SI, Umscheid CA, Bratzler DW, Leas B, Stone EC, Kelz RR, et al. Centers for Disease Control and Prevention Guideline for the Prevention of Surgical Site Infection. *JAMA Surg* 2017; 152 (8): 784-791.

[3] Ban KA, Minei JP, Laronga C, Harbrecht BG, Jensen EH, Fry DE, et al. American College of Surgeons and Surgical Infection Society: surgical site infection guidelines, 2016 update. *J Am Coll Surg* 2017; 224 (1): 59-74.

[4] Culebras JM. Malnutrition in the twenty-fi rst century: an epidemic aff ecting surgical outcome. *Surg Infect (Larchmt)* 2013, 14: 237–43.

[5] Bernabeu-Wittel M, Jadad A, Moreno-Gavino L, et al. Peeking through the cracks: an assessment of the prevalence, clinical characteristics and health-

related quality of life (HRQoL) of people with polypathology in a hospital setting. *Arch Gerontol Geriatr* 2009.

[6] Charles M, Charlene C, et al. A.S.P.E.N. Clinical Guidelines Nutrition Screening, Assessment, and Intervention in Adults. *Journal of Parenteral and Enteral Nutrition* 2011; 35(1):16-24.

[7] Paul EW, Franco C, David C, et al. American society for enhanced recovery and perioperative quality initiative joint consensus statement on nutrition screening and therapy within a surgical enhanced recovery pathway. *Anesth Analg 2018*; 126(6):1883-1895.

[8] Grass F, Bertrand PC, Schäfer M, et al. Compliance with preoperative oral nutritional supplements in patients at nutritional risk—only a question of will? *Eur J Clin Nutr* 2015; 69:525–529.

[9] Elia M, Normand C, Norman K, Laviano A. A systematic review of the cost and cost effectiveness of using standard oral nutritional supplements in the hospital setting. *Clin Nutr* 2016; 35:370–380.

[10] WHO. Gobal guidelines for the prevention of surgical site infections. *World Health Organization*, Geneva, 2016.

[11] Harbis A, Perdreau S, Vincent-Baudry S, et al. Glycemic and insulinemic meal responses modulate postprandial hepatic and intestinal lipoprotein accumulation in obese, insulin-resistant subjects. *Am J Clin Nutr 2004*; 80:896–902.

[12] Osland E, Yunus RM, Khan S, Memon MA. Early versus traditional postoperative feeding in patients undergoing resectional gastrointestinal surgery: a meta-analysis. *JPEN J Parenter Enteral Nutr* 2011; 35:473–487.

[13] Webster J, Osborne S. Preoperative bathing or showering with skin antiseptics to prevent surgical site infection. *Cochrane Database of Systematic Reviews* 2015, Issue 2. Art. No.: CD004985.

[14] Chlebicki MP, Safdar N, O'Horo JC, Maki DG. Preoperative chlorhexidine shower of bath for prevention of surgical site infection: a meta-analysis. *Am J Infect Control.* 2013; 41(2):167-173.

[15] Tanner J, Norrie P, Melen K. Preoperative hair removal to reduce surgical site infection. *Cochrane Database of Systematic Reviews* 2011, Issue 11. Art. No.: CD004122. DOI: 10.1002/14651858.CD004122.pub4.

[16] Ruiz-Tovar J, Badia JM Prevention of surgical site infection in abdominal surgery. A critical review of the evidence. *Cir Esp.*2014;92(4):223-231.

[17] Phippen M, Papanier M. *Patient care during operative and invasive procedures.* Philadelphia: WB Saunders Co, 2000.

[18] Zapata-Copete J, Aguilera-Mosquera S, García-Perdomo HA. Antibiotic prophylaxis in breast reduction surgery: a systematic review and meta-analysis. *J Plast Reconstr Aesthet Surg.* 2017;70(12):1689-1695.

[19] Simons MP, Smietanski M, Bonjer HJ, Bittner R, Miserez M, Aufenacker TJ, et al. International guidelines for groin hernia management. *Hernia.* 2018;22(1):1-165.

[20] Vamvakidis K, Rellos K, Tsourma M, Christoforides C, Anastasiou E, Zorbas KA, et al. Antibiotic prophylaxis for clean neck surgery. *Ann R Coll Surg Engl.* 2017;99(5):410-412.

[21] Ruangsin S, Laohawiriyakamol S, Sunpaweravong S, Mahatta-nobon S, The efficacy of cefazolin in reducing surgical site infection in laparoscopic cholecystectomy: a prospective randomized double-blind controlled trial. *Surg Endosc.* 2015; 29(4):874-881.

[22] Alexander JW, Solomkin JS, Edwards MJ, Updated recommenda-tions for control of surgical site infections. *Ann Surg.* 2011; 253(6):1082-1093.

[23] Peppard WJ, Eberle DG, Kugler NW, Mabrey DM, Weigelt JA, Association between Pre-Operative Cefazolin Dose and Surgical Site Infection in Obese Patients. *Surg Infect (Larchmt).* 2017; 18(4):485-490.

[24] Sidhwa F, Itani K. Skin preparation before surgery: Options and Evidence. *Surg Infect (Larchmt).* 2015;16(1):14-23.

[25] Anderson DJ, Podgorny K, Berríos-Torres SI, Bratzler DW, Dellinger EP, Greene L, et al. Strategies to prevent surgical site infections in acute care hospitals: 2014 update. *Infect Control Hosp Epidemiol.* 2014;35(6):605-627.

[26] Webster J, Alghamdi A. Use of plastic adhesive drapes during surgery for preventing surgical site infection. *Cochrane Database Syst Rev.* 2015(4):CD006353.

[27] Leaper DJ, Edmiston CE. World Health Organization: global guidelines for the prevention of surgical site infection. *J Hosp Infect.* 2017;95(2):135-6.

[28] Horiuchi T, Tanishima H, Tamagawa K, Matsuura I, Nakai H, Shouno Y, et al. Randomized, controlled investigation of the anti-infective properties of the Alexis retractor/protector of incision sites. *J Trauma.* 2007;62(1):212-5.

[29] Reid K, Pockney P, Draganic B, Smith SR. Barrier wound protection decreases surgical site infection in open elective colorectal surgery: a randomized clinical trial. *Dis Colon Rectum.* 2010;53(10):1374-80.

[30] Wilkes RP, Kilpad DV, Zhao Y, Kazala R, McNulty A. Closed incision management with negative pressure wound therapy (CIM): biomechanics. *Surg Innov.* 2012; 19:67-75.

[31] Jansen-Winkeln B, Niebisch S, Scheuermann U, Gockel I, Mehdorn M. Biomechanical Effects of Incisional Negative Wound Pressure Dressing: An Ex Vivo Model Using Human and Porcine Abdominal Walls. *Biomed Res Int.;* 2018:7058461.

[32] Streubel PN, Stinner DJ, Obremskey WT: Use of negative-pressure wound therapy in orthopaedic trauma. *J Am Acad Orthop Surg* 2012; 20(9):564-574.

[33] Turtiainen J, Hakala T, Hakkarainen T, Karhukorpi J. The impact of surgical wound bacterial colonization on the incidence of surgical site infection after lower limb vascular surgery: A prospective observational study. *Eur J Vasc Endovasc Surg* 2014; 47:411–417.

Chapter 4

Microbiology and Treatment of Nosocomial Site Infection

Andrés García Marín[1,2,*], MD, PhD and Mercedes Pérez-López[3]

[1]Department of Surgery, Hospital de Hellín, Albacete, Spain
[2]University Alfonso X El Sabio, Madrid, Spain
[3]Department of Nursery,
Hospital San Vicente del Raspeig, Alicante, Spain

Abstract

Nosocomial infections, also known as Healthcare-associated infections or Hospital-acquired infections are infections that are not present at the time of admission, occurring from 48 hours after admission to 10 days after hospital discharge. The main microorganism involved in surgical site infection were *Staphylococcus. aureus, coagulase-negative staphylococcus, Enterococcus spp., Escherichia coli, Pseudomonas aeruginosa, Enterobacter, Klebsiella pneumoniae*, with a high prevalence of multidrug-resistant pathogens such as *Methicillin-resistant Staphylococcus aureus*, Extended-spectrum beta-lactamase-producing Enterobacteriaceae, fungi and viruses. Management of HAI is based on source control, antibiotics and fluid resuscitation with vasoactive drugs if it is necessary.

---

[*] Corresponding Author's E-mail: agmarin1980@gmail.com.

In: Nosocomial Infection in Abdominal Surgery
Editors: Jaime Ruiz-Tovar and Andrés García Marín
ISBN: 978-1-68507-603-0
© 2022 Nova Science Publishers, Inc.

Keywords: nosocomial site infection, hospital-acquired infection, healthcare-acquired infection, surgical site infection, microbiology, multidrug-resistant pathogens, antibiotics

Introduction

Nosocomial infections, also known as Healthcare-associated infections or Hospital-acquired infections (HAI) are infections that are not present at the time of admission, occurring from 48 hours after admission to 10 days after hospital discharge. HAI include central line-associated bloodstream infections, catheter-associated urinary tract infections, surgical site infections (SSI), pneumonia and Clostridium difficile infections [1, 2].

According to the Center for Disease Control and Prevention, about 4% of hospitalized patients suffer at least one of HAI, whereas World Health Organization estimates that 15% of hospitalized patients suffer any HAI, being the most frequent pneumonia, SSI and gastrointestinal infections. As well as, in the United States HAI are the sixth leading cause of death [1, 2].

The risk for HAI depends on patients (higher risk includes immunosuppression, older age, length of hospital stay, comorbidities, invasive procedures, recent antibiotic therapy), prevalence of pathogens within the community and infection control policy. Recently, preoperative 25-hydroxy vitamin D levels has been strongly associated with postoperative SSI [1-4].

The pathogens can be acquired from hospital workers, patients or hospital facilities. The recent COVID-19 pandemic has taught us an important forgotten lesson, the reduction of SSI with the implementation of hygienic measures (hand washing) and the systematic use of personal protective equipment (masking, gloves) among healthcare workers and patients. A California study involving 37033 hospital patient days reported that following implementation of a COVID-19 infection control bundle, rates of many multidrug-resistant pathogens decreased significantly including a 41% decrease in methicillin-resistant *Staphylococcus aureus* (MRSA), a 21% decrease in extended-spectrum β-lactamase-producing Enterobacteriaceae and an 80% decrease in *vancomycin-resistant enterococci* (VRE) [5, 6].

HAI are associated with increased length of hospital stay and mortality in hospitalized patients [1, 2, 6-10].

The aim of the present chapter is to describe the microbiology and the treatment of nosocomial SSI.

Microbiology

Involved microorganisms can be gram-positive cocci (*Staphylococcus spp.*, *Streptococcus spp.* and, less frequently, *Enterococcus spp.*), gram-negative bacilli (*Escherichia coli*, *Proteus* spp., *Klebsiella* spp., *Pseudomonas* spp.) and anaerobes (*Bacteroides* spp., *Clostridium* spp.). According to the CDC, the most frequent pathogens involved in HAI were *Clostridium difficile, Staphylococcus aureus, Klebsiella* spp. and *Escherichia coli*. However, according to the National Healthcare Safety Network, the main microorganisms involved in SSI were *Staphylococcus. aureus, coagulase-negative staphylococcus, Enterococcus faaecalis and faecium, Escherichia coli, Pseudomonas aeruginosa, Enterobacter, Klebsiella pneumoniae*. One of the most important problem is the higher prevalence of multidrug-resistant pathogens particularly in the intensive care unit with reduced susceptibility to standard antibiotic regimens, such as MRSA, *coagulase-negative staphylococci*, VRE, *extended-spectrum beta-lactamase-producing Enterobacteriaceae, quinolone-resistant Escherichia coli*, non-fermenting gram-negative bacteria (*Pseudomonas aeruginosa, Acinetobacter baumannii* and *Stenotrophomonas maltophilia*), fungi (*Candida* spp. [mainly *Candida albicans, Candida parapsilosis* and *Candida tropicalis*], *Aspergillus* spp.). Candida infections arise from patient's endogenous microflora whereas Aspergillus infections are caused by inhalation of fungal spores from contaminated air during construction or renovation of health care facility) and viruses (5% of HAI), which can be transmitted through hand-mouth, respiratory route and fecal-oral route. Hepatitis B and C are commonly transmitted through unsafe injection practices. Factors predisposing to multidrug-resistant pathogens include corticosteroid use, recent exposure to broad-spectrum antibiotics (less than 3 months), underlying conditions such as liver disease, pulmonary disease, organ transplantation and a length of hospitalization greater than 5 days [1, 2, 8-22].

Treatment

Management of HAI is based on source control, antibiotics and fluid resuscitation with vasoactive drugs if it is necessary [6, 7].

Source control is the first key to a successful treatment, which can be performed as soon as possible. It includes drainage of abscesses, debridement of infected necrotic tissues, removal of potentially infected devices, abdominal compartment cleansing and measures to control contamination and restore normal gastrointestinal anatomy and function (suture, bowel resection, ostomy, appendectomy, cholecystectomy, etc.). The least invasive approach that achieves definitive source control or enough control to allow resolution of the inflammatory response and organ dysfunction should be performed. Source control failure should be considered if there is a progressive organ dysfunction within the first 24-48 hours after source control, if there is no clinical improvement in organ dysfunction 48 hours or more after source control, or if there are persistent signs of inflammation 5-7 days after source control. Source control can be completed by a single intervention, but many studies have reported that failure to obtain adequate source control is one of the most strong factors associated with an adverse outcome, including death. Routine cultures should be obtained to identify underlying microorganisms [6-10].

The selection and timing of initiation of antibiotics are critical. International guidelines for management of sepsis and septic shock (survival sepsis campaign) recommend appropriate routine microbiological cultures (including blood) be obtained before starting antimicrobial therapy in patients with suspected sepsis or septic shock if doing so results in no substantial delay in the start of antimicrobials. Intravenous antibiotics should be initiated as soon as possible after recognition and within 1 hour for both sepsis and septic shock. Also, guidelines recommend empiric broad-spectrum therapy with one or more antimicrobials for patients with sepsis or septic shock to cover all likely pathogens and the spectrum should be narrowed once pathogens and their sensitivities are established and clinical improvement is noted. Selection of antibiotics are based on comorbidities, recent known infection or colonization with specific pathogens, previous antibiotics within the previous three months, site of infection, susceptibility patterns of pathogens in the community and hospital. Inadequate empirical antibiotic therapy was associated with a higher mortality rate [6-15].

The recommended antibiotic regimen is based on piperacillin-tazobactam, imipenem-cilastatin and meropenem. In patients with β-lactam allergies, the recommended antibiotics are tigecycline, aztreonam/ aminoglycosides (gentamicin, tobramycin) plus metronidazole plus vancomycin/linezolid. If *Pseudomonas aeruginosa* are suspected, aminoglycoside, ceftazidime or cefepime should be added [6-10].

Risk factors for invasive candidiasis include previous surgical procedure, broad-spectrum antimicrobial therapy, pancreatitis, use of parenteral nutrition, invasive catheters, comorbidities such as diabetes mellitus, heart disease, renal failure, immunosuppression and multiple sites of colonization with *Candida spp*. Mortality rates range from 20 to 64%, especially if the initiation of treatment is delayed. The problem is the difficulty to prove invasive candidiasis, since the definitive criteria based on histological analysis is not useful in daily management. Therefore, antifungal therapy initiation is based on clinical scores. Candida score ≥ 3 (surgery 1 point; parenteral nutrition 1 point; multiple sites of colonization 1 point; severe sepsis 2 points) involves initiation of antifungal therapy. Echinocandin (anidulafungin, caspofungin or micafungin) is recommended in severe sepsis/septic shock/previous treatment with fluconazole/previous colonization by fluconazole resistant *Candida spp*. (*C. glabrata* and *C. krusei*). Fluconazole is recommended in absence of severe sepsis/septic shock/previous treatment with fluconazole [6-14].

Antimicrobial Doses

a) Imipenem-cilastatin: 0.5 - 1 gr/6-8 hours. Dose adjustment is necessary in chronic renal insufficiency according to creatinine clearance:
   i) 41-70 ml/min: 750 mg/8 hours.
   ii) 21-40 ml/min: 500 mg/6 hours.
   iii) 6-20 ml/min: 500 mg/12 hours.
b) Meropenem: 0.5 - 1 gr/6-8 hours. Dose adjustment is necessary in chronic renal insufficiency according to creatinine clearance:
   i) 26-50 ml/min: 1 g/12 hours.
   ii) < 25 ml/min: 500 mg/12 hours.
c) Piperacillin-tazobactam: 4 g/500 mg/horas. Dose adjustment is necessary in chronic renal insufficiency according to creatinine clearance:
   i) 20-40 ml/min: 2 g/250 mg/6 hours.
   ii) < 20 ml/min: 2 g/250 mg/8 hours.
d) Tigecycline: 100 mg initial loading dose and 50 mg/12 hours. Dose adjustment is not required in chronic renal or liver insufficiency (Child A-B). Decrease maintenance dose to 25 mg/12 hours in patients with chronic liver insufficiency Child C without change in initial loading dose. Broad-spectrum antibiotic without coverage for Proteus spp., Pseudomonas spp. and Providentia spp.
e) Vancomycin: 1 g/12 hours. Dose adjustment is necessary in chronic renal insufficiency according to creatinine clearance:

      i) 25-50 ml/min: 1 g/24 hours.
      ii) < 25 ml/min: 1 g/48 hours.
f) Linezolid: 600 mg/12 hours. Dose adjustment is not required in chronic renal or liver insufficiency.
g) Aminoglycosides: gentamicin/tobramycin 5 mg/kg of total weight whereas amykacin 15-20 mg/kg of total weight. Continuous monitoring is necessary to check peak and valley levels. Recommended peak and valley levels are 5-10 µg/ml and < 2 µg/ml with gentamicin/tobramycin respectively whereas 20-30 µg/ml and 1-8 µg/ml with amykacin.
h) Aztreonam: 1-2 g/8 hours. Dose adjustment is necessary in chronic renal insufficiency according to creatinine clearance:
      i) 10-30 ml/min: 50% reduction of doses, after initial doses of 1-2 g.
      ii) < 10 ml/min: 75% reduction of doses, after initial doses of 1-2 g.
i) Metronidazole: 500 mg/8 hours. Dose adjustment is necessary in chronic renal insufficiency according to creatinine clearance: < 10 ml/min: 50% reduction of dose. Decrease dose to 500 mg/12-24 hours in patients with chronic liver insufficiency Child A-C.
j) Ceftazidime: 1-2 g/8 hours. Dose adjustment is necessary in chronic renal insufficiency according to creatinine clearance:
      i) 31-50 ml/min: 1 g/12 hours.
      ii) 16-30 ml/min: 1 g/24 hours.
      iii) 6-15 ml/min: 0.5 g/24 hours.
      iv) < 5 ml/min: 0.5 g/48 hours.
k) Fluconazole: 400 mg/24 hours. Dose adjustment is necessary in chronic renal insufficiency according to creatinine clearance:
      i) 10-50 ml/min: 50% reduction of doses or 400 mg/48 hours.
      ii) < 10 ml/min: 75% reduction of doses or 400 mg/72 hours.
l) Equinocandine:
      i) Caspofungin: 70 mg initial loading dose and 50 mg/24 hours. Dose adjustment is necessary in moderate chronic liver insufficiency: 35 mg/24 hours.
      ii) Anidulafungin: 200 mg initial loading dose and 100 mg/24 hours. Dose adjustment is not required in chronic renal or liver insufficiency.
      iii) Micafungin: 100 mg/24 hours. Dose adjustment is not required in chronic renal or liver insufficiency [6, 7, 18].

Conclusion

Nosocomial infections are infections that are not present at the time of admission. Involved microorganisms can be gram-positive cocci, gram-negative bacilli and anaerobes, with a higher prevalence of multidrug-resistant pathogens particularly in the intensive care unit with reduced susceptibility to standard antibiotic regimens, such as MRSA, c*oagulase-negative staphylococci*, VRE, *extended-spectrum beta-lactamase-producing Enterobacteriaceae, quinolone-resistant Escherichia coli*, non-fermenting gram-negative bacteria (*Pseudomonas aeruginosa, Acinetobacter baumannii* and *Stenotrophomonas maltophilia*), fungi (*Candida* spp., *Aspergillus* spp.). The management of nosocomial infections are based on source control, antibiotics and fluid resuscitation with vasoactive drugs if it is necessary.

References

[1] Khan H A, Baig F A, Mehboob R. Nosocomial infections: epidemiology, prevention, control and surveillance. *Asian Pac. J. Trop. Biomed.*, 2017;7:478-82.

[2] Liu J Y, Dikter J K. Nosocomial infections: a history of Hospital-acquired infections. *Gastrointest. Endosc. Clin. N. Am.*, 2020;30: 637-52.

[3] Abdehgah A G, Monshizadeh A, Tehrani M M, Afhami S, Molavi B, Jafari M, et al. Relationship between preoperative 25-hydroxy vitamin D and surgical site infection. *J. Surg. Res.*, 2020; 245: 338-43.

[4] Laviano E, Sánchez M, González-Nicolás M T, Palacian M P, López J, Gilaberte Y, et al. Surgical site infection in hepatobiliary surgery patients and its relationship with serum vitamin D concentration. *Cir. Esp.*, 2020; 98: 456-64.

[5] Cole J, Barnard E. The impact of the COVID-10 pandemic on healthcare acquired infections with multidrug resistant organisms. *Am. J. Infect. Control*, 2021; 49: 653-4.

[6] Losurdo P, Paiano L, Samardzic N, Germani P, Bernardi L, Borelli M, et al. Impact of lockdown for SARS-CoV-2 (COVD-19) on surgical site infection rates: a monocentric observational cohort study. *Updates Surg.*, 2020; 14: 1-9.

[7] Levy M M, Evans L E, Rhodes A. The surviving sepsis campaign bundle: 2018 update. *Intensive Care Med.*, 2018; 44: 925-8.

[8] Rhodes A, Evans L E, Alhazzani W, Levy M M, Antonelli M, Ferrer R, et al. Surviving Sepsis Campaign: International Guidelines for Management of Sepsis and Septic Shock: 2016. *Intensive Care Med.*, 2017; 43: 304-77.

[9] Membrilla-Fernández E, Sancho-Insenser J J, Girvent-Montllor M, Álvarez-Lerma F, Sitges-Serra A. Secondary Peritonitis Spanish Study Group. Effect of initial empiric antibiotic therapy combined with control of the infection focus on the prognosis of patients with secondary peritonitis. *Surg. Infect. (Larchmt)*, 2014; 15: 806-14.

[10] Montravers P, Blot S, Dimopoulos G, Eckmann C, Eggimann P, Guirao X, et al. Therapeutic management of peritonitis: a comprehensive guide for intensivists. *Intensive Care Med.*, 2016; 42: 1234-7.

[11] Rattan R, Allen C J, Sawyer R G, Askari R, Banton K L, Coimbra R, et al. Percutaneously drained intra-abdominal infections do not require longer duration of antimicrobial therapy. *J. Trauma Acute Care Surg.*, 2016; 81: 108-12.

[12] Sartelly M, Catena F, Anasaloni L, Coccolini F, Di Saverio S, Griffiths E A. Duration of antimicrobial therapy in treating complicated intra-abdominal infections: a comprehensive review. *Surg. Infect. (Larchmt)*, 2016; 17: 9-12.

[13] Sawyer R G, Claridge J A, Nathens A B, Rotstein O K, Duane T M, Evans H L, et al. Trial of short-course antimicrobial therapy for intraabdominal infection. *N. Engl. J. Med.*, 2015; 372: 1996-2005.

[14] Syue L S, Chen Y H, Ko W C, Hsueh P R. New drugs for the treatment of complicated intra-abdominal infections in the era of increasing antimicrobial resistance. *Int. J. Antimicrob. Agents.*, 2016; 47: 250-8.

[15] Turza K C, Politano A D, Rosenberg L H, Riccio L M, McLeod M, Sawyer R G. De-escalation of antibiotics does not increase mortality in critically ill surgical patients. *Surg. Infect. (Larchmt)*, 2016; 17: 48-52.

[16] Sharma R, Eun-Park T, Moy S. Ceftazidime-avibactam: a novel cephalosporin/beta-lactamase inhibitor combination for the treatment of resistant gram-negative organisms. *Clin. Ther.*, 2016; 38: 431-44.

[17] Montravers P, Lepape A, Dubreuil L, Gauzit R, Pean Y, Benchimol D, et al. Clinical and microbiological profiles of community-acquired and nosocomial intra-abdominal infections: results of the French prospective, observational EBIIA study. *J. Antimicrob. Chemother.*, 2009; 63: 785-94.

[18] Maseda E, Suárez de la Rica A., Anillo V, Tamayo E, García-Bernedo C A, Ramasco F, et al. Procalcitonin-guided therapy may reduce length of antibiotic treatment in intensive care unit patients with secondary peritonitis: a multicenter retrospective study. *J. Crit. Care*, 2015; 30: 537-42.

[19] Mazuski J, Tessier J, May A K, Sawyer R G, Nadler E P, Rosengart M R, et al. The Surgical Infection Society Revised Guidelines on the Management of Intra-Abdominal Infection. *Surg. Infect. (Larchmt)*, 2017; 18: 1-76.
[20] Strobel R, Kreis M, Lauscher J C. Surgical site infections-Prevention and treatment strategies. *Chirurg.*, 2021; 92: 385-94.
[21] Cai Y, Lo J J, Venkatachalam I, Kwa A L, Tambyah P A, Hsu L Y, et al. The impact of healthcare associated infections on mortality and length of stay in Singapore. A time-varying analysis. *Infect. Control Hosp. Epidemiol.*, 202; 41: 1315-20.
[22] Augustin P, Tanaka S, Tran-Dinh A, Ribeiro L P, Arapis K, Grall N, et al. Outcome and adequacy of empirical antibiotherapy in post-operative peritonitis: a retrospective study. *Surg. Infect. (Larchmt)*, 2020; 21: 284-92.

Chapter 5

Nosocomial Urinary Tract Infection

Ana Sánchez-Mozo[1,*] and Héctor Aguado-López[2]
[1]Department of General and Digestive Surgery,
Complejo Hospitalario Universitario de Albacete, Albacete, Spain.
[2]Department of General and Digestive Surgery,
Hospital de Hellín, Hellín, Albacete, Spain

Abstract

Hospital-acquired infections (HAI) or nosocomial infections are a major cause of morbidity, mortality and economic cost in healthcare systems worldwide. Nosocomial urinary tract infections (NUTIs) are one of the most frequent HAI (20-30%). Risk factors are prolonged use of urinary catheters, urological surgery and genitourinary manipulations. Usually the bacterial focus is endogenous and the most commonly isolated microorganisms are Gram-negative bacteria (66%), especially Escherichia coli and Pseudomonas. Symptoms (fever, dysuria, pyuria) and urinary cultures (typically, the growth of 100.000 or more organisms per milliliter of urine) have been the standard means for diagnosing urinary tract infections. When NUTI is diagnosed, it should be treated with antimicrobial therapy, regardless of whether the patient has urinary catheter or not. Asymptomatic bacteriuria does not necessarily need antimicrobial therapy (could be treated with remove or exchange urinary catheter). Resistance to common antibiotics for urinary pathogens is currently a topic of concern, so it's very important for prevention, especially of catheter-associated urinary tract infections (CAUTI).

---

[*] Corresponding Author's E-mail: anasanchezmozo@gmail.com.

In: Nosocomial Infection in Abdominal Surgery
Editors: Jaime Ruiz-Tovar and Andrés García Marín
ISBN: 978-1-68507-603-0
© 2022 Nova Science Publishers, Inc.

Keywords: nosocomial infections, urinary tract infections, catheter-associated urinary tract infections

Introduction

Nosocomial urinary tract infection (NUTI) is defined like urinary tract infection (UTI) is acquired in any healthcare institution or, more generally, when it is related to patient management.

NUTI are between 20-30% of hospital-acquired infections (HAI). In the past, NUTI was the most frequent HAI, but currently, others HAI (respiratory tract infections, surgical site infections) are more frequent than NUTI.

HAIs are a major cause of morbidity, mortality and economic cost in healthcare systems worldwide, so that it's very important for prevention. In NUTIs, the most important prevention is catheter-associated urinary tract infections (CAUTI); it's the most frequent NUTI.

This chapter aims to highlight the current urological knowledge about definition, epidemiology and risk factors, pathogenesis, etiology, clinical features, diagnosis, prevention and treatment of NUTIs.

Methods

Definition

UTI is a commonly used term, which has the advantage to immediately describe the site of infection. Introduced in 1957, UTI definition was based on the bacterial count. Kass developed the concept of significant bacteriuria (>100000 colony-forming units per milliliter – CFU/mL) in the context of pyelonephritis in pregnancy. Although this concept introduced quantitative microbiology into the diagnosis of infectious diseases, it has recently become clear that there is no fixed bacterial count that is indicative of significant bacteriuria, which can be applied to all kinds of UTIs and in all circumstances [1-2]. Following the guides, it can be defined as [3]:

Urinary Tract Infection -- UTI.
UTI is defined as the colonization and subsequent multiplication of microorganisms in the urinary system (usually sterile), associated with symptoms (or not) that can be specific or non-specific.

Nosocomial Urinary Tract Infection – NUTI
Like it was said, NUTI is defined when UTI is acquired in any healthcare institution or, more generally, when it is related to patient management. About 80% of NUTIs are CAUTIs.

Catheter Associated Urinary Tract Infection -- CAUTI
CAUTI is defined as any UTI related to the presence of a urinary catheter. It can be NUTI or in the community. Usually CAUTIs occur in healthcare institutions (NUTI) but they are also associated with patients who have a home urinary catheter.

No Catheter Associated Urinary Tract Infection -- No-CAUTI
No-CAUTI is defined as any UTI that is not related to the presence of a urinary catheter. It can be NUTI or in the community. Usually No-CAUTIs occur in the community, most of them are symptomatic. In this group are cystitis, urethritis, prostatitis and pyelonephritis.

Asymptomatic Bacteriuria -- ASB
Also called "colonization of the urinary tract", ASB is defined as the presence of one (or several) microorganisms in the urinary tract without clinical manifestations. ASB is associated with the presence of a urinary catheter that has been colonized in most cases.

Epidemiology and Risk Factors

NUTI are between 20-30% of HAI. In the past, NUTI was the most frequent HAI, but currently, other HAIs (respiratory tract infections, surgical site infections) are more frequent than NUTI. Sometimes, according to the studies, NUTI is considered the second or third HAI in frequency.

The most important risk factors are prolonged use of urinary catheters, urological surgery and genitourinary manipulations. These factors allow the

NUTIs to be classified in catheter-associated urinary infections (CAUTIs) or no catheter-associated urinary infections (No-CAUTIs) [4]:

- About 80% of NUTIs are CAUTIs. The wrong use of urinary catheters increases CAUTIs. Many urinary catheters are unnecessary in hospitalized patients and when the catheters are needed, they are used too long. It's estimated the indication for urinary catheter was not considered adequate in 8% of cases and continuation of bladder catheterization was considered unnecessary in 32%. Multivariate analyses have emphasized that the duration of catheterization is the most important risk factor in the development of CAUTIs.
- About 10-20% of NUTIs are related to urological surgery and genitourinary manipulations (No-CAUTIs). These infections are frequent in patients with gynecological pathology.

There are some groups of patients who are more risk of develop NUTIs, highlighting three groups:

- Intensive care unit (ICU) patients are an important risk group for developing NUTIs. These patients have more aggressive diseases and a higher risk of immunosuppression.
- Pregnant patients are another important risk group for developing NUTIs. These patients present genitourinary manipulations and need a urinary catheter when a cesarean is performed.
- Other groups of risk patients are older patients. Currently, ederly patients represent the largest percentage of hospital admissions and their immune system is weaker than other patients. They also have a higher risk of having a urinary catheter and bladder incontinence.

Other risk factors are: diabetes mellitus, female gender, impaired renal function, colonization of the drainage bag, poor quality of catheter care and immunosuppressed patients (transplant patients, oncology patients) [5].

Pathogenesis

In normal conditions, the urinary tract has innate defense mechanisms that prevent colonization of the urinary bladder. These include the length of the urethra and urination. On the other hand, the urinary tract secretes adhesion inhibitors of bacteria and various mucopolysaccharides. Furthermore, pH and urinary osmolarity inhibit the bacterial growth.

In the catheterized patient, the catheter bulb prevents complete emptying of the catheter, leaving residual urine. Urinary catheterization has been observed interferes with these defense mechanisms.

The source of microorganisms causing CAUTI can be endogenous, typically via meatal, rectal, or vaginal colonization, or exogenous, such as via contaminated equipment or healthcare staff's hands [6].

- Endogenous source: The most frequent source. It can happen by 2 mechanisms:
  o During catheter insertion, especially, in elderly patients with urethral colonization by uropathogens
  o Exoluminal via. The microorganisms come from the flora of the patient's intestinal tract or vaginal, colonize the perineum and ascend through the space between the catheter and the urethra.
- Exogenous source: It is more infrequent; It can happen intraluminal via, through the lumen of the catheter, either by breaking the closed drainage system at the connections or ascending from the collection bag. In this case as a result of transmission of contaminated equipment or healthcare staff's hands.

Two factors are essential in the pathogenesis of CAUTI: adhesion and the capacity for biofilm formation, which depends on both the microorganism and the type of urinary catheter. Silicone or hydrogel-coated catheters are more resistant to bacteria attachment than rubber or latex. Additionally, silicone catheters cause less urethral inflammation and urethral stricture.

Once attached, the bacteria will secrete a series of polysaccharides that in a few days will form an extracellular matrix called glucocalyx or biofilm. The formation of biofilms by urinary pathogens on the surface of the catheter and drainage system occurs universally with prolonged duration of catheterization. Inside the biofilm, bacterial growth is slower (probably due to a lack of oxygen and nutrients) and the bacteria become more resistant to antimicrobials.

Over time, the urinary catheter becomes colonized with microorganisms living in the state within the biofilm, making them resistant to antimicrobials and host defenses virtually impossible to eradicate without removing the catheter.

Certain microorganisms have the ability to hydrolyze urea (by the action of bacterial ureases) and lead to the formation of crystal deposits, which will occlude the catheter, favoring the development of bacteremia; this happens from a pH of 6.7 or higher.

On the other hand, bacterial motility may be a pathogenic factor to consider, thanks to the presence of fimbriae or pili that have the ability to adhere to specific uroepithelial receptors [7].

Etiology

The most common pathogens of NUTIs are the patient's own colonic flora [3, 5]. Gram-negative pathogens predominate (60%), especially *Escherichia coli* (30-40% NUTIs). Other gram-negative organisms are *Klebsiella pneumoniae, Pseudomonas aeruginosa, Proteus mirabilis, Acinetobacter baumannii, Enterobacter cloacae* and *Serratia spp*. Among gram-positive pathogens stand out *Enterococcus* (15%) and to a lesser extent *Staphylococcus*. Another common pathogen is *Candida spp.* (10-15%) and overall 10% are polymicrobial NUTIs.

The most common pathogens of No-CAUTIs is *Escherichia coli* (45%) followed by *Enterococcus* (15%) and *Klebsiella pneumoniae* (15%).

The most common pathogens of CAUTIs is *Escherichia coli* (30-35%) followed by *Klebsiella pneumoniae* (15%), *Candida* spp. (15%) and *Pseudomonas aeruginosa* (10%).

Candida spp. and *Pseudomonas aeruginosa* are important in patients admitted to the ICU and patients with risk factors because they appear significantly more frequently as agents in urosepsis.

Clinical

The clinical presentation of UTI is variable and with nonspecific signs and symptoms [8].

Fever (>38°C) is the most frequent symptom associated with UTI. Usually fever appears in patients with a urinary catheter and ICU patients, although it can occur in other UTIs

Other signs and symptoms are suprapubic pain at palpation or tenderness, costovertebral angle pain or tenderness, urinary urgency, urinary frequency and dysuria. These signs and symtoms suggest a urological problem although they are not exclusive, especially, costovertebral angle pain and suprapubic pain or tenderness.

ASB doesn't present any symptoms, therefore, it should be suspected in patients with urinary catheters or patients with altered level of consciousness. In this case, the clinical will not help the diagnosis.

Diagnosis

Under normal conditions, urine is sterile, although it can become contaminated as it passes through the urethra. When there is a microbial contamination of the urinary system, with or without disease, the easiest way to detect it is to look for the presence of these microorganisms in urine [7].

For diagnosis of UTI, we can use optical microscopes (Gram stain, pyuria) and urinary cultures.

- Gram stain: Bacteriuria is considered to exist when it is detected, by gram staining, one or more bacteria in uncentrifuged urine. Gram stain may be useful for empirical treatment, especially in serious and critical patients.
- Pyuria is considered to exist when more than 10 leukocytes per field are detected in urine centrifuged at 2,000 rpm for 5 minutes. The presence of pyuria has little predictive value.
- Urinary cultures have been the standard means for diagnosing UTI. The standard cutoff has been the growth of 100.000 or more organisms per milliliter of urine (colony-forming units per milliliter – CFU/mL). This number was originally based on studies of symptomatic patients with cystitis, and not hospitalized patients with infections related to urinary catheter. Nonetheless, this remains the number used to diagnose the presence of NUTIs, although in recent years it has been considered as positive cultures with 10.000 CFU/mL associated with systemic signs and symptoms.

Generally, as described above, ASB is defined as the presence of a positive urine culture (100.000 or more CFU/mL) without symptoms. A patient with a symptomatic UTI must show one or more symptoms or findings, additional to a positive urine culture.

The degree of pyuria does not allow differentiation between the patient with symptomatic UTI or ASB. However, the absence of pyuria in a patient with urinary symptoms should suggest another diagnosis than UTI.

Following the Center for Disease Control and Prevention (CDC), the Infectious Diseases Society of America (IDSA) and the European Society for Clinical Microbiology and Infectious Diseases (ESCMID) for the diagnosis of NUTI, symptomatic UTI, ASB, and CAUTIs as: [3, 9-10]

NUTI

NUTI is defined as any UTI (symptomatic UTI, ASB, CAUTI) acquired in any health institution.

Symptomatic UTI

Symptomatic UTI is defined like one of the following two criteria:

1. One of the following symptoms: fever (>38°C), frequent bladder urgency, dysuria or suprapubic pain at palpation and a positive urinary culture with ≥100.000 CFU/mL urine with two or less bacterial species
2. Two of the following symptoms: fever (>38°C), frequent bladder urgency, dysuria or syprapubic pain at palpation and one of the following findings:
   (a) Evidence of leukocyte-esterase and/or nitrate.
   (b) Pyuria (≥10 leukocytes/mm3 or ≥3 leukocytes/high power field at x400 magnifications of uncentrifuged urine).
   (c) Microscopic evidence of pathogen in Gram-stain of uncentrifuged urine.
   (d) Two urinary cultures with an identical uropathogen ≥100.000 CFU/mL from correctly obtained specimens;
   (e) Pure culture with ≤100.000 CFU/mL after appropriate antibiotic treatment.

ASB

To define ABS, urinary culture is mandatory and the following criteria must be met:

1. A urinary catheter was in place for more than seven days prior to the urinary specimen and the patient had no fever (<38°C), frequent bladder urge, dysuria or suprapubic pain on palpation. The urinary culture, however, must be positive with ≥100.000 CFU/mL with two or less bacterial species.
2. The patient had no urinary catheter in place for seven days prior to the first of two urinary specimens with ≥100.000 CFU/mL urine of an identical uropathogen (not more than two distinct species) and the patient neither shows fever (>38°C), nor frequency, dysuria or suprapubic pain.
3. If clinical signs cannot be ascertained, (sedated patients), an infection is probable when uropathogens are detected in a significant number (catheter urine ≥100.000 CFU/mL; any detection of uropathogens in bladder aspirate), with not more than two distinct species cultured.

CAUTI

For a patient to be classified as having a CAUTI, the patient must meet all 3 of the following criteria:

1. Patient had an indwelling urinary catheter that had been in place for more than 2 days on the date of event (day of device placement -- day 1) and was either:
   (a) Present for any portion of the calendar day on the date of event
   or
   (b) Removed the day before the date of event
2. Patient has at least 1 of the following signs or symptoms: Fever (>38°C), suprapubic tenderness, costovertebral angle pain or tenderness, urinary urgency or urinary frequency, dysuria.
3. Patient has a urine culture with no more than 2 species of organisms identified, at least 1 of which is a bacterium of ≥100.000 CFU/mL.

All criteria must occur during the infection window period.

Prevention

The best way to avoid and treatment NUTIs is to prevent them. Like it was said in chapter "Epidemiology and Risk factors", many urinary catheters are unnecessary in hospitalized patients and when the catheters are needed, they are used too long. The risk for bacteriuria with catheterization is 5% to 10% per day and the risk increases to almost 100% after 30 days of catheterization. About 70% of CAUTIs can be prevented by following the guidelines recommended, which would reduce morbidity, mortality and economic cost in healthcare systems.

There are guidelines for preventing NUTIs, especially CAUTIs. These guidelines show key points to help prevent them. The most important key points are: [11, 12, 13]

All Hospitalized Patients Need a Urinary Catheter?

All hospitalized patients do not need a urinary catheter.

The patients are admitted in ICU and operative patients need urinary catheter but the patients are admitted on ward usually do not need it and should be avoid their use in patients for management of incontinence.

Alternatives like intermittent catheterization should be considered in adults with spinal cord injury and children with myelomeningocele and neurogenic bladder to reduce the risk of urinary tract deterioration.

How Long should the Catheter Remain?

The duration of catheterization should be minimal

Minimize urinary catheter use and duration in all patients, particularly when the mortality risk may be higher due to catheterization, such as in the elderly and in patients with severe illness. In non-urological surgeries recommend removing the catheter within the first 24 hours.

When long-term catheters are required they should be changed in intervals adapted to the individual patient, however, there is no evidence for the exact intervals of changing catheters.

How Should the Catheter be Placed?
Which Catheter Should be Used?

The objective is to prevent or delay biofilm formation in the urinary catheter.

It's recommended to perform the aseptic insertion of the urinary catheter (sterile gloves, chlorhexidine in the urinary meatus) but it is not recommended installation of antiseptic solutions into urinary drainage bags and urinary catheter.

It's recommended to maintain a closed drainage system and it's suggested to use urinary catheter systems with preconnected and sealed catheter-tubing junctions.

Hydrophilic catheters are recommended to standard catheters for patients requiring intermittent catheterization

Antibiotic Prophylaxis Should be Used to Prevent NUTIs in Patients Who Need a Urinary Catheter?

Antibiotic prophylaxis should not be used to prevent NUTIs in catheterized patients

The wrong use of antibiotics increases antibacterial resistance. Antibiotics resistance is one of the medical war in century XXI

Treatment

Treatment of NUTIs needs to be considered separately for patients with ASB and for those with symptomatic urinary tract infection.

In general, ASB in catheterized patients should not be treated with antibiotics. Usually, it's enough to remove the urinary catheter to solve ASB. Guidelines recommended use antibiotics in a few cases:

- For patients undergoing urological surgery.
- For patients who have a high risk of serious infectious complications (immunosuppressed).
- Control other HAI due to a particularly virulent organism.
- For infections originating by strains causing a high incidence of bacteremia.

Treatment of symptomatic NUTIs is more straightforward. The most frequent symptom is fever. Other symptoms are dysuria, pyuria and suprapubic pain. When symptomatic NUTIs are diagnosed, empiric antibiotics should be started, based on knowledge of the local bacterial ecology, and then tailored based on definitive culture and susceptibility results. There is no consensus on the duration of treatment, the guides recommended use antibiotics individually; patient response and clinical should be used to determine the duration of the antibiotic course [13].

In community-acquired urinary tract infections, usually use penicillin's (ampicillin, amoxicillin), 1st generation cephalosporin (cefazolin, cephalexin), quinolones (ciprofloxacin, levofloxacin), trimethoprim/sulfamethoxazole or fosfomycin.

The problem is these antibiotics develop resistance more frequently in NUTIs The choice of antibiotic may be complicated. The bacteria acquire resistance to multiple antibacterial drugs mainly through horizontal transfer of mobile genetic elements such as transposons or plasmids.

The gram-negative bacilli ESBL-positive (Extended Spectrum Beta Lactamase) strains are resistant to all extended beta-lactam antibacterial drugs such as cephalosporins. Around 15% are ESBL-positive and their frequency is often underestimated. MRSA-positive (Methicillin-resistant Staphylococcus aureus) is another resistance mechanism of some gram-positive cocci.

For example, *Escherichia coli* is resistant to 1st and 2rd generation cephalosporins in 30-40% and to fluoroquinolones in 45-50% of the cases of NUTIs. There is more resistance in patients admitted on ICU and CAUTIs compared with patients admitted on ward and No-CAUTIs.

Treatment of *Candida spp.* is special. Usually, *Candida spp.* is infrequent in patients admitted to ward and these patients rarely present symptomatic candiduria. As with other ABS, asymptomatic candiduria doesn´t need pharmacologic therapy. Pharmacologic therapy with an antifungal agent should generally be limited to patients with symptomatic candiduria after confirmation of the infection from a second urine sample. Unfortunately, the critically ill patient is the one most likely to have candiduria, and the one least likely to be able to complain of symptoms. Furthermore, this is the patient most likely to suffer a poor outcome if a necessary treatment is retarded. In general, candiduria should be treated in patients admitted in ICU, symptomatic candiduria and immunosuppressed patients.

For empirical therapy of NUTI (without risk factors) some options are amoxicillin/clavulanic, ciprofloxacine or cefotaxime. If initial therapy fails, piperacillin/tazobactam cefepime, imipenem or gentamicin (monotherapy or combination) associated or not with fluconazole are good options.

For empirical therapy of a severe NUTI (urosepsis, ICU patients) broad-spectrum antibiotics should be used: cefepime + gentamicin (or amikacin), imipenem, piperacillin/tazobactam, vancomycin (combinated) associated or not with fluconazole are good options. In this case, it must use antibiotics against ESBL, MRSA and Pseudomonas [14].

Conclusion

Nosocomial urinary tract infections are one of the most frequent hospital-acquired infections (20-30%). Risk factors are prolonged use of urinary catheters, urological surgery and genitourinary manipulations. Usually the bacterial focus is endogenous and the most commonly isolated microorganisms are Gram-negative bacteria (66%), especially Escherichia coli and Pseudomonas. Fever, dysuria and pyuria associated urinary cultures have been the standard means for diagnosing urinary tract infections. When nosocomial urinary tract infection is diagnosed, it should be treated with antimicrobial therapy. Asymptomatic bacteriuria does not necessarily need antimicrobial therapy (could be treated with remove or exchange urinary catheter). Resistance to common antibiotics for urinary pathogens is currently a topic of concern, so it's very important for prevention, especially of catheter-associated urinary tract infections.

References

[1] Kass, EH. Bacteriuria and the diagnosis of infections of the urinary tract; with observations on the use of methionine as a urinary antiseptic. *AMA Arch Intern Med.*, 1957, 100(5), 709-714.
[2] Kass, EH. Bacteriuria and pyelonephritis of pregnancy. *Arch Intern Med.*, 1960 Feb, 105, 194-8.
[3] Horan, TC; Andrus, M; Dudeck, MA. CDC/NHSN surveillance definition of health care associated infection and criteria for specific types of infections in the acute care setting. *Am J Infect Control*, 2012, 36 (5).
[4] Chenowth, CE; Saint, S. Urinary tract infections. *Infect Dis Clin North Am.*, 2011, 25, 103–15.

[5] Nicolle, LE. Urinay catheter-associated infections. *Infect Dis Clin North Am.*, 2012, 26, 13–27.
[6] Iacovelli, V; Gaziev, G; Topazio, L; Bove, P; Vespasiani, G; Finazzi Agrò, E. Nosocomial urinary tract infections: A review. *Urologia.*, 2014, 81(4), 222-227.
[7] Pigrau, C. Infecciones del tracto urinario nosocomiales [Nocosomial urinary tract infections]. *Enferm Infecc Microbiol Clin.*, 2013, 31(9), 614-624.
[8] Bouza, E; San Juan, R; Muñoz, P; Voss, A; Kluytmans, J. Co-operative Group of the European Study Group on Nosocomial Infections. A European perspective on nosocomial urinary tract infections II. Report on incidence, clinical characteristics and outcome (ESGNI-004 study). European Study Group on Nosocomial Infection. *Clin Microbiol Infect.*, 2001 Oct, 7(10), 532-42.
[9] Rubin, USE; Andriole, VT; Davis, RJ; Stamm, WE. Evaluation of new anti-infective drugs for the treatment of UTI. *Clin Infect Dis.*, 1992, 15, 216.
[10] Rubin, UH SE; Andriole, VT; Davis, RJ; Stamm, WE. with a modification by a European Working Party (Norrby SR). *General guidelines for the evaluation of new anti-infective drugs for the treatment of urinary tract infection*. The European Society of Clinical Microbiology and Infectious diseases, Taukirchen, Germany, 1993, p. 240-310
[11] Gould, CV; Umscheid, CA; Agarwal, RK; et al. Guideline for prevention of catheter associated urinary tract infections. *Infect Control Hosp Epidemiol*, 2010, 31, 319–26.
[12] Tenke, P; Kovacs, B; Bjerklund Johansen, TE; et al. European and Asian guidelines on management and prevention of catheter-associated urinary tract infections. *Int J Antimicrob Agents*, 2008, 31(Suppl 1), S68–78.
[13] Hooton, TM; Bradley, SF; Cardenas, DD; et al. Diagnosis, prevention, and treatment of catheter-associated urinary tract infection in adults: 2009 International Clinical Practice Guidelines from the Infectious Diseases Society of America. *Clin Infect Dis*, 2010, 50, 625.
[14] Weiner, LM; Webb, AK; Limbago, B; et al. Antimicrobial-Resistant Pathogens Associated With Healthcare-Associated Infections: Summary of Data Reported to the National Healthcare Safety Network at the Centers for Disease Control and Prevention, 2011-2014. *Infect Control Hosp Epidemiol*, 2016, 37, 1288.

Chapter 6

Nosocomial Respiratory Tract Infection

Francisco Javier Ruescas García[1] and Celia Pérez Parra[2,*]

[1]Department of General and Digestive Surgery,
Hospital de Hellín, Albacete, Spain
[2]Departament of Obstetrics and Gynecology,
Hospital de Almansa, Spain

Abstract

Despite advances in antibiotic treatment, improvement in supportive therapy and preventive measures, nosocomial pneumonia (NP) continues to be a major cause of morbidity and mortality, especially in critically ill surgical patients, with an estimated incidence between 5 and 15 per 1000 hospitalized patients. The most frequently implicated pathogens in NP are *Enterobacteriaceae, Staphylococcus aureus, Pseudomonas aeruginosa, Haemophilus influenzae, and Acinetobacter baumannii*. We must know both the risk factors for NP and factors that increase the possibility of infection by multidrug-resistant pathogens (MDR), to apply the appropriate preventive measures and an early and adequate antibiotic treatment, since a delay in the initiation of it has demonstrated an increase in mortality, and overtreatment leads to an increased risk of selection of MDR pathogens.

Keywords: respiratory infections, pneumonia, nosocomial infections, abdominal surgery.

---

* Corresponding Author's E-mail: ruescas4@hotmail.com.

In: Nosocomial Infection in Abdominal Surgery
Editors: Jaime Ruiz-Tovar and Andrés García Marín
ISBN: 978-1-68507-603-0
© 2022 Nova Science Publishers, Inc.

Introduction

Nosocomial Pneumonia (NP) remains a major cause of morbidity and mortality despite advances in antimicrobial therapy, improved supportive therapy modalities, and the use of a wide range of preventive measures. Surgical patients are especially sensitive to NP and it is mainly associated with patients requiring mechanical ventilation. NP is defined as a pneumonia that affects any patient who was hospitalized in an acute care hospital for two or more days within 90 days after infection; resided in a nursing home or long-term care facility; received recent intravenous antibiotic therapy, chemotherapy, or wound care within the last 30 days of current infection; or attended a hospital or hemodialysis clinic. Hospital associated pneumonia (HAP) is defined as pneumonia occurring 48 hours or more after admission, which was not incubating at the time of admission. Ventilator associate pneumonia (VAP) is defined as pneumonia that appears 48 hours after endotracheal intubation and is the most common nosocomial infection in the ICU in surgery patients.

Epidemiology

Incidence

The incidence of NP is estimated to be between 5 and 15 cases per 1000 hospital admissions, the main predisposing factor being the presence of mechanical ventilation, which increases the risk of PN between 6 and 20 times, so that VAP represents 80% of patients of the total of NP cases. The incidence of VAP ranges from 1.9 to 3.8 cases per 1000 ventilator days in the United States, exceeding 18 cases per 1000 days of intubation in Europe, as reported by Koulenti et al., in a prospective observational multicenter study. The incidence of VAP increases with the duration of mechanical ventilation, at a rate of 3% per day during the first 5 days, 2% per day during days 5 to 10 and 1% per day from day 10.

Mortality associated with VAP has been estimated to be between 20% and 50%, with a directly attributable mortality of 18% as described by Magill et al., in a meta-analysis. It was associated with bacteremia, especially *Pseudomonas aeruginosa* or *Acinetobacter* species, medical rather than surgical conditions, and ineffective antibiotic therapy.

Etiology

NP can be caused by a broad spectrum of bacterial pathogens, being due to polymycobial infection in more than 32% of VAPs, especially in patients with acute respiratory distress syndrome (ARDS). They are rarely due to viral or fungal infections in immunocompetent patients. The most frequently isolated pathogens in VAP are Enterobacteriaceae, *Staphylococcus aureus, Pseudomonas aeruginosa, Haemophilus influenzae,* and *Acinetobacter baumannii.* In contrast, *enterococci, viridanns streptococci,* and *coagulase-negative staphylococci* are hardly identifiable as a cause of respiratory dysfunction.

The frequency of MDR pathogens that cause NP may vary by hospital, with the following identified as risk factors:

- Use of intravenous antibiotics in the past 90 days.
- ≥5 days of hospitalization before the appearance of VAP.
- Septic shock at the time of VAP.
- ARDS before VAP.
- Acute renal replacement therapy before VAP.

Pathogeny

For NP to occur, an imbalance is required between the host's defenses (both mechanical, humorous and cellular) and the liability of the microorganism for colonization and invasion of the lower respiratory tract, in favor of the latter to establish infection. The main sources of pathogens for NP include the use of sanitary devices, the environment (air, water, equipment, and fomites), and the spread of microorganisms between the patient and staff or other patients. The main routes of bacterial entry to the lower respiratory tract are the aspiration of oropharyngeal pathogens and the leakage of secretions through the cuff of the endotracheal tube. In the case of PAVs, the infected biofilm in the endotracheal tube and subsequent embolization to the distal airways can be an important source of pathogen entry. However, direct inhalation or inoculation of pathogens into the lower respiratory tract, hematogenous spread from infected intravenous catheters, and bacterial translocation of the lumens of the gastrointestinal tract do not appear to be a common cause of lung infection.

Risk Factors

Endotracheal intubation and mechanical ventilation is the highest risk factor for NP, multiplying the risk 6 to 20 times.

Among the rest of the risk factors for PN described in the literature, the following stand out:

- Age: extremes of life (<2 and ≥ 60 years)
- Prolonged hospitalization (≥ 14 days)
- Acute respiratory distress syndrome (ARDS)
- Chronic obstructive disease
- Coma or impaired consciousness
- Malnutrition (albumin <2.2 g / dl)
- Burns and trauma
- Recent head, neck, thoracic or upper abdominal surgery
- Blood transfusion
- One or more organs failure
- Supine position and gastric aspirate
- Sinusitis, tracheobronchitis
- Immunosuppression, corticosteroid treatment

Classification

VAP can be classified as early-onset pneumonia, when it appears within the first 4 days of endotracheal intubation, or late-onset when it appears at 5 days or later. Early-onset VAP is frequently due to aspiration of gastric contents, has a better prognosis, and is usually due to antibiotic-sensitive pathogens such as methicillin-sensitive *S. aureus, Streptococus pneumoniae*, and *Haemophilus influenzae*. Late presentation VAPs are more frequently caused by multidrug-resistant pathogens (MDRs) such as *P. auriginosa* or *Acinetobacter* and are associated with higher mortality. However, patients with early-onset VAP who have received previous antibiotics or who have been previously hospitalized in the last 90 days are at increased risk of colonization and infection with MDR pathogens and should be treated similarly to patients with late-onset VAP.

Diagnosis

The diagnosis of VAP is complicated, since non-infectious processes such as congestive heart failure, atelectasis, ARDS or pulmonary embolism can coexist, which could cause alterations in the chest radiograph and in gas exchange. In contrast, immunosuppressed patients may present with pneumonia without a cough, fever, sputum, or leukocytosis. If false positive diagnoses occur, patients are exposed to antibiotic overtreatment, with the consequent increased risk of infection by MDR pathogens. On the contrary, if it is not diagnosed in time, a delay in the starting of treatment increases mortality.

The most common findings of nosocomial pneumonia are worsening oxygenation, purulent sputum, the development of fever, and leukocytosis, along with a new or progressive pulmonary radiographic infiltration picture. When fever, leukocytosis, purulent sputum develop, and a positive sputum culture or tracheal aspirate without new pulmonary infiltration, the diagnosis of nosocomial tracheobronchitis should be considered.

Clinical criteria such as those of the Center for Disease Control and Prevention for the diagnosis of VAP that do not require identification of the pathogen causing the infection, underestimate the incidence of VAP, compared to histological or microbiological data. The diagnostic criteria for radiographic infiltration and at least one clinical feature (fever, leukocytosis, or purulent tracheal secretions) have high sensitivity but low specificity for VAP. However, combinations of signs and symptoms can increase specificity. Fábregas et al., in a study in which the diagnostic standard was histology plus positive microbiological cultures of postmortem lung samples, the presence of thoracic infiltrates, plus two of three clinical criteria resulted in 69% sensitivity and 75% specificity for the diagnosis of VAP.

The Clinical Pulmonary Infection Scale (CPIS) incorporates clinical, radiographic, and microbiological criteria (Table 1), up to a maximum of 12 points. A value greater than 6 points indicates a high probability of VAP. However, the specificity is not greater than that of the clinical picture alone when compared with cultures of samples by bronchoalveolar lavage or with protected brushing. In the previously named study of Fábregas et al., CPIS had a sensitivity of 77% and a specificity of 42%.

Table 1. Clinical Pulmonary Infection Score (CPIS)

Clinical Parameter	Points
Teperature (°C)	
36.5-38.4	0
38.5-38.9	1
≥39 or ≤36	2
Blood leukocytes (x $10^3/mm^3$)	
4 – 11	0
<4 or >11	1
Band forms ≥50%	2
Tracheal secretions	
Absent	0
Nonpurulent	1
Purulent	2
Oxygenation: PaO_2/FiO_2 (mm Hg)	
>240 or ARDS	0
≤240 and no evidence ARDS	2
Infiltrate on pulmonary radiography	
None	0
Diffuse or patchy	1
Localized	2
PATHOGENIC BACTERIA ON TRACHEAL-ASPIRATE CULTURE	
RARE, LIGHT QUALITY OR NOGROWTH	0
MODERATE OR HEAVY QUANTITY	1
ALSO SEEN ON GRAM´S STAIN	2

PaO_2: arterial partial pressure of oxygen. FiO_2: fraction of inspired oxygen. ARDS: acute respiratory distress syndrome.

Given the low specificity of traditional diagnoses, culture of lower respiratory samples is recommended before starting antibiotic treatment to minimize false negative results. The collection of samples for culture can be invasive such as blind brushing and bronchoalveolar lavage (they collect samples by fiberoptic bronchoscopy and allow direct vision of the airways) or non-invasive such as endotracheal suction aspiration, the blind telescopic catheter connected, blind protected brushing and brocoalveolar mini flush. Their analysis can be semi-quantitative (referred to in ordinal categories as light, moderate or intense) or quantitative (in colony-forming units per milliliter of aliquot).

Bronchoscopic specimen collection techniques are more specific than blind techniques and both are superior to endotracheal suction aspiration. Shorr et al., in a meta-analysis of randomized trials comparing patients with

VAP approached by obtaining invasive and non-invasive samples, analyzed with quantitative cultures, it suggested a survival advantage in the invasive approach but not significantly.

Procalcitonin is a precursor to calcitonin that is constitutively secreted by C cells of the thyroid gland and K cells of the lung. It may be useful in the diagnosis of PN, but it has not been shown to be useful for the management of antibiotic treatment in critical patients with VAP, since it did not improve survival and did cause organ-related damage and prolonged admission to the unit of intensive care in a randomized trial published by Jensen et al.

Prevention

As previously described, endotracheal intubation and mechanical ventilation are the main risk factor for PN. Therefore, we must reduce its use to the minimum possible, and if necessary, maintain mechanical ventilation for the essential time. An alternative to reduce the endotracheal intubation rate is noninvasive positive pressure ventilation, whenever it is possible. Orotracheal intubation has been shown to be superior to nasotracheal, since the former reduces the risk by 50% by reducing the risk of nosocomial sinusitis and possibly VAP.

After intubation, the measures to prevent VAP must be aimed at preventing the aspiration of gastric contents, for this the use of sedatives and muscle relaxants must be limited, which limit coughing. We also have to maintain an endotracheal cuff pressure above 20 mmHg, in addition, new materials have been developed for the endotracheal cuff and technologies that facilitate its adherence to the trachea. Subglottic aspiration greatly reduces the risk of VAP.

Elevation of the head 30-45° has also been shown to be effective in preventing VAP in the supine position, especially during enteral feeding, since it reduces the risk of aspiration. Another measure to reduce the risk of gastroesophageal reflux and aspiration, and with it the appearance of VAP, is post-pyloric feeding.

Pharmacological measures aimed at reducing the incidence of VAP lead to the prophylaxis of stress ulcers and selective digestive decontamination with antibiotics (topical or systemic) or antiseptics. Although selective decontamination of the digestive tract with antibiotics reduces NP, its routine prophylactic use is discouraged, especially in hospital settings where there are high levels of antibiotic resistance.

Blood transfusion has been related to the risk of VAP in surgery patients, being described as an independent risk factor. Hébert et al., as early as 1999 in a multicenter, ramdomized and prospective study, it showed that in patients without acute coronary disease or unstable angina, expect a hemoglobin level of 7.0 g/dl instead of a level of 9.0 g/dl before starting transfusion is at least as effective or possibly superior, leading to less transfusion and no adverse effect on outcome. Earley et al., achieved a significant reduction in the incidence of VAP (8.1% vs 0.8%, $p = 0.002$) in a surgical ICU after an anemia management protocol that resulted in a reduction in blood transfusions.

Antibiotic Treatment

For an adequate treatment of NP and VAP we must emphasize the importance of applying an early and appropriate antibiotic treatment in adequate doses, avoiding antibiotic overtreatment by de-escalation of the initial antibiotic therapy, based on microbiological cultures and the clinical response of the patient and shortening the duration of treatment to the minimum effective period to decrease the risk of selection for MDR pathogens. The delay in initiating adequate antibiotic treatment has been associated with increased mortality. In addition, we must take into account local microbiological data when adapting treatment recommendations to any specific clinical setting.

We can differentiate two groups of patients, the first one is patients with NP of early presentation and without risk factors for MDR pathogens (mentioned previously), they do not require broad spectrum therapy, and a second group that we must treat with broad therapy spectrum, because they present late-onset pneumonia or risk factors for infection with MDR pathogens.

Empirical treatment of patients with severe PAH or VAP requires the use of antibiotics at optimal doses to ensure maximum efficacy. Initial treatment should be administered to all patients intravenously, with a switch to oral/enteral therapy in selected patients with a good clinical response and a functional intestinal tract.

Monotherapy should be used when it is possible, especially in patients without risk factors for MDR bacteria, because combination therapy increases the cost of treatment and exposes patients to unnecessary antibiotics, thus increasing the risk of MDR pathogens and complications such as nephrotoxicity. Monotherapy is also the standard when the pathogen causing

NP is gram positive, including methicillin-resistant Staphylococcus aereus (MRSA).

If after the start of antibiotic treatment the lower respiratory tract cultures are absent or growth below the predetermined threshold and the patient does not show deterioration, the antimicrobial treatment can be stopped. When a susceptible pathogen grows in the culture, the treatment should be desiccated to a narrow-spectrum antimicrobial for that pathogen. On the contrary, if a multi-resistant pathogen appears in the crop, we can continue with the same spectrum or broaden it if necessary to combat the pathogen.

In patients receiving an initially appropriate antibiotic regimen, efforts should be made to shorten the duration of treatment from the traditional 14 to 21 days to short periods such as 7 days, provided that the etiological pathogen is not P. aeruginosa and that the patient has a good clinical response to infection, being equally effective, as demonstrated by Chastre et al., in a randomized multicenter study. In patients with less severe VAP or less likely to have VAP with CPIS ≤ 6, a three-day course of antibiotics may be enaugh.

The Infectious Diseases Society of America and the American Thoracic Society recommend including coverage for *S. aureus, Pseudomonas aeruginosa*, and other gram-negative bacilli in all empirical regimens suspected of VAP. They also suggest including an active agent against MRSA (vancomycin or linezolid) for the empirical treatment of suspected VAP only in patients, a risk factor for antimicrobial resistance, in patients treated in units where >10% -20% of *S aureus* isolates are resistant to methicillin or in patients treated in units where the prevalence of MRSA is unknown. In the remaining cases, they recommend including an active antibiotic against Methicillin-sensitive
S. aureus (piperacillin-tazobactam, cefepime, levofloxacin, imipenem or meropenem). Regarding antipseudomonal treatment, they recommend using two antibiotics with different mechanisms of action for the empirical treatment of suspected VAP only in patients who present a risk factor for antimicrobial resistance, in patients in units where > 10% of the gram-isolated negatives are resistant to an agent that is considered for monotherapy or in patients treated in an ICU where no local rates of antimicrobial susceptibility are available. If none of these factors are present, they recommend treatment with an active antibiotic against *P. aeruginosa*.

Conclusion

The main risk factor for PN is endotracheal intubation and mechanical ventilation, therefore we must reduce their use to the minimum possible, using alternatives such as non-invasive positive pressure ventilation. Once PN is established, we must apply an early and appropriate antibiotic treatment in adequate doses, based on microbiological cultures and the patient's clinical response, thus shortening the duration of treatment to the minimum effective period.

References

Adair CG, Gorman SP, Feron BM, Byers LM, Jones DS, Goldsmith CE, Moore JE, Kerr JR, Curran MD, Hogg G, Webb CH, McCarthy GJ, Milligan KR. Implications of endotracheal tube biofilm for ventilator-associated pneumonia. *Intensive Care Med.* 1999 Oct;25(10):1072-6. doi: 10.1007/s001340051014. PMID: 10551961.

American Thoracic Society; Infectious Diseases Society of America. Guidelines for the management of adults with hospital-acquired, ventilator-associated, and healthcare-associated pneumonia. *Am J Respir Crit Care Med.* 2005 Feb 15;171(4):388-416. doi: 10.1164/rccm.200405-644ST. PMID: 15699079.

Beardsley JR, Williamson JC, Johnson JW, Ohl CA, Karchmer TB, Bowton DL. Using local microbiologic data to develop institution-specific guidelines for the treatment of hospital-acquired pneumonia. *Chest.* 2006 Sep;130(3):787-93. doi: 10.1378/chest.130.3.787. PMID: 16963676.

Berton DC, Kalil AC, Teixeira PJ. Quantitative versus qualitative cultures of respiratory secretions for clinical outcomes in patients with ventilator-associated pneumonia. *Cochrane Database Syst Rev.* 2014 Oct 30;(10):CD006482. doi: 10.1002/14651858.CD006482.pub4. PMID: 25354013.

Celis R, Torres A, Gatell JM, Almela M, Rodríguez-Roisin R, Agustí-Vidal A. Nosocomial pneumonia. A multivariate analysis of risk and prognosis. *Chest.* 1988 Feb;93(2):318-24. doi: 10.1378/chest.93.2.318. PMID: 3338299.

Chastre J, Fagon JY. Ventilator-associated pneumonia. *Am J Respir Crit Care Med.* 2002 Apr 1;165(7):867-903. doi: 10.1164/ajrccm.165.7.2105078. PMID: 11934711.

Chastre J, Wolff M, Fagon JY, Chevret S, Thomas F, Wermert D, Clementi E, Gonzalez J, Jusserand D, Asfar P, Perrin D, Fieux F, Aubas S; PneumA Trial Group. Comparison of 8 vs 15 days of antibiotic therapy for ventilator-associated pneumonia in adults: a randomized trial. *JAMA*. 2003 Nov 19;290(19):2588-98. doi: 10.1001/jama.290.19.2588. PMID: 14625336.

Cook D, De Jonghe B, Brochard L, Brun-Buisson C. Influence of airway management on ventilator-associated pneumonia: evidence from randomized trials. *JAMA*. 1998 Mar 11;279(10):781-7. doi: 10.1001/jama.279. 10.781. Erratum in: *JAMA* 1999 Jun 9;281(22):2089. PMID: 9508156.

Cook DJ, Walter SD, Cook RJ, Griffith LE, Guyatt GH, Leasa D, Jaeschke RZ, Brun-Buisson C. Incidence of and risk factors for ventilator-associated pneumonia in critically ill patients. *Ann Intern Med*. 1998 Sep 15;129(6):433-40. doi: 10.7326/0003-4819-129-6-199809150-00002. PMID: 9735080.

Earley AS, Gracias VH, Haut E, Sicoutris CP, Wiebe DJ, Reilly PM, Schwab CW. Anemia management program reduces transfusion volumes, incidence of ventilator-associated pneumonia, and cost in trauma patients. *J Trauma*. 2006 Jul;61(1):1-5; discussion 5-7. doi: 10.1097/01.ta.0000225925.53583.27. PMID: 16832243.

Fàbregas N, Ewig S, Torres A, El-Ebiary M, Ramirez J, de La Bellacasa JP, Bauer T, Cabello H. Clinical diagnosis of ventilator associated pneumonia revisited: comparative validation using immediate post-mortem lung biopsies. *Thorax*. 1999 Oct;54(10):867-73. doi: 10.1136/thx.54.10.867. PMID: 10491448; PMCID: PMC1745365.

Hébert PC, Wells G, Blajchman MA, Marshall J, Martin C, Pagliarello G, Tweeddale M, Schweitzer I, Yetisir E. A multicenter, randomized, controlled clinical trial of transfusion requirements in critical care. Transfusion Requirements in Critical Care Investigators, Canadian Critical Care Trials Group. *N Engl J Med*. 1999 Feb 11;340(6):409-17. doi: 10.1056/NEJM 199902113400601. Erratum in: N Engl J Med 1999 Apr 1;340(13):1056. PMID: 9971864.

Heyland DK, Cook DJ, Griffith L, Keenan SP, Brun-Buisson C. The attributable morbidity and mortality of ventilator-associated pneumonia in the critically ill patient. The Canadian Critical Trials Group. *Am J Respir Crit Care Med*. 1999 Apr;159(4 Pt 1):1249-56. doi: 10.1164/ajrccm.159.4.9807050. PMID: 10194173.

Holzapfel L, Chastang C, Demingeon G, Bohe J, Piralla B, Coupry A. A randomized study assessing the systematic search for maxillary sinusitis in nasotracheally mechanically ventilated patients. Influence of nosocomial maxillary sinusitis on the occurrence of ventilator-associated pneumonia. *Am J Respir Crit Care Med*. 1999 Mar;159(3):695-701. doi: 10.1164/ajrccm. 159.3.9712076. PMID: 10051239.

Jensen JU, Hein L, Lundgren B, Bestle MH, Mohr TT, Andersen MH, Thornberg KJ, Løken J, Steensen M, Fox Z, Tousi H, Søe-Jensen P, Lauritsen AØ, Strange D, Petersen PL, Reiter N, Hestad S, Thormar K, Fjeldborg P, Larsen

KM, Drenck NE, Ostergaard C, Kjær J, Grarup J, Lundgren JD; Procalcitonin And Survival Study (PASS) Group. Procalcitonin-guided interventions against infections to increase early appropriate antibiotics and improve survival in the intensive care unit: a randomized trial. *Crit Care Med.* 2011 Sep;39(9):2048-58. doi: 10.1097/CCM.0b013e31821e8791. PMID: 21572 328.

Kalil AC, Metersky ML, Klompas M, Muscedere J, Sweeney DA, Palmer LB, Napolitano LM, O'Grady NP, Bartlett JG, Carratalà J, El Solh AA, Ewig S, Fey PD, File TM Jr, Restrepo MI, Roberts JA, Waterer GW, Cruse P, Knight SL, Brozek JL. Management of Adults With Hospital-acquired and Ventilator-associated Pneumonia: 2016 Clinical Practice Guidelines by the Infectious Diseases Society of America and the American Thoracic Society. *Clin Infect Dis.* 2016 Sep 1;63(5):e61-e111. doi: 10.1093/cid/ciw353. Epub 2016 Jul 14. Erratum in: *Clin Infect Dis.* 2017 May 1;64(9):1298. Erratum in: *Clin Infect Dis.* 2017 Oct 15;65(8):1435. Erratum in: *Clin Infect Dis.* 2017 Nov 29;65(12):2161. PMID: 27418577; PMCID: PMC4981759.

Kollef MH, Kollef KE. Antibiotic utilization and outcomes for patients with clinically suspected ventilator-associated pneumonia and negative quantitative BAL culture results. *Chest.* 2005 Oct;128(4):2706-13. doi: 10.1378/chest.128.4.2706. PMID: 16236946.

Kollef MH, Skubas NJ, Sundt TM. A randomized clinical trial of continuous aspiration of subglottic secretions in cardiac surgery patients. *Chest.* 1999 Nov;116(5):1339-46. doi: 10.1378/chest.116.5.1339. PMID: 10559097.

Koulenti D, Tsigou E, Rello J. Nosocomial pneumonia in 27 ICUs in Europe: perspectives from the EU-VAP/CAP study. *Eur J Clin Microbiol Infect Dis.* 2017 Nov;36(11):1999-2006. doi: 10.1007/s10096-016-2703-z. Epub 2016 Jun 10. PMID: 27287765.

Kunac A, Sifri ZC, Mohr AM, Horng H, Lavery RF, Livingston DH. Bacteremia and ventilator-associated pneumonia: a marker for contemporaneous extra-pulmonic infection. *Surg Infect (Larchmt).* 2014 Apr;15(2):77-83. doi: 10.1089/sur.2012.030. Epub 2013 Nov 5. PMID: 24192306.

Kuti EL, Patel AA, Coleman CI. Impact of inappropriate antibiotic therapy on mortality in patients with ventilator-associated pneumonia and blood stream infection: a meta-analysis. *J Crit Care.* 2008 Mar;23(1):91-100. doi: 10.1016/j.jcrc.2007.08.007. PMID: 18359426.

Melsen WG, Rovers MM, Groenwold RH, Bergmans DC, Camus C, Bauer TT, Hanisch EW, Klarin B, Koeman M, Krueger WA, Lacherade JC, Lorente L, Memish ZA, Morrow LE, Nardi G, van Nieuwenhoven CA, O'Keefe GE, Nakos G, Scannapieco FA, Seguin P, Staudinger T, Topeli A, Ferrer M, Bonten MJ. Attributable mortality of ventilator-associated pneumonia: a meta-analysis of individual patient data from randomised prevention studies.

Lancet Infect Dis. 2013 Aug;13(8):665-71. doi: 10.1016/S1473-3099(13)70081-1. Epub 2013 Apr 25. PMID: 23622939.

Muscedere J, Rewa O, McKechnie K, Jiang X, Laporta D, Heyland DK. Subglottic secretion drainage for the prevention of ventilator-associated pneumonia: a systematic review and meta-analysis. *Crit Care Med.* 2011 Aug;39(8):1985-91. doi: 10.1097/CCM.0b013e318218a4d9. PMID: 21478738.

Pieracci FM, Barie PS. Strategies in the prevention and management of ventilator-associated pneumonia. *Am Surg.* 2007 May;73(5):419-32. PMID: 17520992.

Pugin J, Auckenthaler R, Mili N, Janssens JP, Lew PD, Suter PM. Diagnosis of ventilator-associated pneumonia by bacteriologic analysis of bronchoscopic and nonbronchoscopic "blind" bronchoalveolar lavage fluid. *Am Rev Respir Dis.* 1991 May;143(5 Pt 1):1121-9. doi: 10.1164/ajrccm/143.5_Pt_1.1121. PMID: 2024824.

S. Barie, Philip. "Surgical infections and Antibiotic Use." In *Sabinston Textbox of Surgery: The Biológical Basics of Modern Surgical Practice.* Edited by Coutney M. Townsend, Jr, 241-280. Philadelphia: Elsevier, 2017. ISBN978-0-323-40162-7.

Tablan OC, Anderson LJ, Besser R, Bridges C, Hajjeh R; CDC; Healthcare Infection Control Practices Advisory Committee. Guidelines for preventing health-care--associated pneumonia, 2003: recommendations of CDC and the Healthcare Infection Control Practices Advisory Committee. *MMWR Recomm Rep.* 2004 Mar 26;53(RR-3):1-36. PMID: 15048056.

Torres A, Serra-Batlles J, Ros E, Piera C, Puig de la Bellacasa J, Cobos A, Lomeña F, Rodríguez-Roisin R. Pulmonary aspiration of gastric contents in patients receiving mechanical ventilation: the effect of body position. *Ann Intern Med.* 1992 Apr 1;116(7):540-3. doi: 10.7326/0003-4819-116-7-540. PMID: 1543307.

Trouillet JL, Chastre J, Vuagnat A, Joly-Guillou ML, Combaux D, Dombret MC, Gibert C. Ventilator-associated pneumonia caused by potentially drug-resistant bacteria. *Am J Respir Crit Care Med.* 1998 Feb;157(2):531-9. doi: 10.1164/ajrccm.157.2.9705064. PMID: 9476869.

Chapter 7

Vascular Access Infection

Héctor Aguado López[1,*] and Ana Sánchez Mozo[2]

[1]Department of General and Digestive Surgery, Hospital de Hellín, Hellín, Albacete, Spain
[2]Department of General and Digestive Surgery,
Complejo Hospitalario Universitario de Albacete, Albacete, Spain

Abstract

Hospital-acquired infections (HAI) or nosocomial infections are a major cause of morbidity, mortality and economic cost in healthcare systems worldwide. Catheter-related bloodstream infections (CRBSIs) are one of the most frequent HAI (15-30%). All intravascular devices confer a risk of infection, although it is estimated that between 75-90% of CRBSIs occur with Central venous catheters (CVCs). Intensive Care Unit patients and poor catheter care are other risk factors. The most common source of CRBSI is colonization of the catheter by microorganisms from the patient's skin. Gram-positive aerobes bacteria represent two thirds of the CRBSIs (60-70%). Coagulase negative staphylococci is the most frequent group followed by Staphylococcus aureus Gram-positive aerobes, gram-negative bacilli and Candida spp. are the other microorganisms. Symptoms (fever, inflammation or purulence at the catheter insertion site, hemodynamic instability and catheter dysfunction) associated with blood cultures and catheter cultures have been the standard means for diagnosing CRBSI. When CRBSI is suspected, it should be treated with antimicrobial therapy and frequently remove the catheter. It's very important for prevention, because CRBSI

---

[*] Corresponding Author's E-mail: h.aguado.lopez@gmail.com.

In: Nosocomial Infection in Abdominal Surgery
Editors: Jaime Ruiz-Tovar and Andrés García Marín
ISBN: 978-1-68507-603-0
© 2022 Nova Science Publishers, Inc.

is an aggressive infection in severe patients and resistance antibiotics are increasing.

Keywords: catheter-related bloodstream infections, vascular access infections, hospital acquired infections, nosocomial infections

Introduction

Catheter-related bloodstream infections (CRBSIs) also called vascular access infections are among the most frequent hospital acquired infections (HAI). Currently, it estimates that between 15% and 30% of all nosocomial bacteremia are CRBSIs.

Intravascular devices have become an essential component of modern medicine for the administration of medication, intravenous fluids, blood products, parenteral nutrition, hemodialysis and for monitoring hemodynamic status.

The incidence of CRBSIs varies considerably. It depends on the insertion site and duration of catheter placement; the type and the frequency with which the catheters accessed, the experience of the individual who places the catheter, the characteristics of the patient, and the prevention strategies

It is estimated that approximately between 75-90% of CRBSIs occur with Central Vascular Catheters (CVCs), though the role of peripheral intravenous access as causes of bloodstream infection is likely underestimated [1].

This chapter aims to highlight the current knowledge about CBRSIs, especially in prevention and treatment.

Methods

Types of Catheters

There are several types of vascular catheters that can be classified in different ways (mode of insertion, use, size, number of lumens, artery/vein where they are placed, and their risk of associated infections). The most important is the place where they act (central or peripheral) and the vessel where they are placed (artery or vein).

The vascular catheters are: [2-3]

- Peripheral venous catheter (PVC): It´s the most used catheter in patients admitted to ward for the administration of medication and intravenous fluids. Usually inserted in veins of the forearm or hand. Risk local infection.
- Peripheral arterial catheter: It´s used for hemodynamic controls. Usually inserted in the radial artery; can be placed in femoral, axillary, brachial, posterior tibial arteries. Low risk of infections.
- Midline catheter: Inserted via the antecubital fossa into the proximal basilic or cephalic veins; does not enter central veins, peripheral catheters. Little used but present lower risk of local infection than peripheral venous catheter.
- Peripherally inserted central venous catheter (PICC): Inserted into basilic, cephalic, or brachial veins and enter the superior vena cava. These catheters are frequently used (parenteral nutrition) and they have less risk infections than CVC.
- Non-tunnelled central venous catheter It´s the CVC most used for temporary treatments and it can have one or more lights. Percutaneously inserted into central veins (subclavian, internal jugular, or femoral). 90% of bacteremia associated with vascular catheters in ICUs.
- Tunneled (or cuffed) central venous catheter: It´s used for long term treatments (hemodialysis) and it can have one or more lights. Implanted into subclavian, internal jugular, or femoral veins. Low risk of infections.
- Totally implantable central venous catheter: Tunneled beneath skin and have subcutaneous port accessed with a needle; implanted in subclavian or internal jugular vein. It´s used for chemotherapy. Low risk of infections.
- Pulmonary artery catheters (Swan-Ganz catheter): Inserted through a Teflon introducer in a central vein (subclavian, internal jugular, or femoral) to the pulmonary artery. It is used for monitoring for a few days. Low risk infection.
- Central arterial catheter: Catheter generally placed through the femoral artery for filtration procedures or hemodynamic monitoring. High risk of infections
- Umbilical catheters: Used in neonatal patients. They can be placed in the umbilical artery and vein.

The most used vascular catheters are: PVC in patients admitted on ward; non-tunnelled CVC and peripheral artery catheter in ICU patients; PICCs, tunneled CVC and totally implantable CVC for long term treatments.

Although the use of any type of vascular catheter carries a risk of developing an infection, between 75% and 80% of CRBSIs is originated in the CVCs

Epidemiology and Risk Factors

Currently, the incidence of CRBSIs is decreasing, possibly as a result of widespread prevention efforts, although CRBSIs continue to be an important cause of morbidity and mortality worldwide. CRBSI is related to 3 factors: host factors, catheter factors and hospital factors [4].

Host Factors
The most important host factors are chronic illness, immune deficiency (especially neutropenia) and loss of skin integrity (as with burns).

Neutropenic patients are also at high risk for infections. Those with an absolute neutrophil count (polymorphonuclear leukocytes) below 100 cells/mm^3 appear to be at the greatest risk.

Patients hospitalized with burns are at particularly increased risk for HAI, as the necrotic tissue in the burn wounds increases the susceptibility to infection, thermal trauma decreases host resistance, and the body exhibits an inflammatory reaction to these processes.

Other host factors are bone marrow transplantation, chemotherapy, hemodialysis, malnutrition, total parenteral nutrition administration, extremes of age and previous CRBSI [5].

Catheter Factors
All intravascular devices confer a risk of infection, although some carry greater risk than others. The most important catheter factors are type and anatomic location of the catheter.

The risk according to the type of the catheter is probably the most important factor of all. Central arterial catheter is the catheter with the highest risk, although they are only used for monitoring and their use is not very frequent.

CVC is the catheter that causes more CRBSIs (75%-80%) but not all CVCs have the same risk. Non-tunneled CVCs have more risk than tunneled CVCs and tunneled CVCs have more risk than totally implantable CVCs [6].

Peripheral venous catheters have low risk infection but they are placed very frequently, they cause a significant percentage of CRBSIs. PICC is the catheter with lowest risk.

The anatomic location of the catheter is another risk factor. It has to differentiate between upper and lower extremities, there is more risk in lower extremities than upper extremities. It is also necessary to differentiate in which central vessel they are placed, there is more risk in femoral or internal jugular placement than subclavian placement

Others catheter factors are duration of catheterization (although there is no indication for routine line changing based on number of catheter days), type of catheter material, conditions of insertion, skill of the catheter inserter, multiple-lumen catheter and catheter-site care [7].

Hospital Factors

It has two important hospital factors: Intensive Care Unit (ICU) patients and the hospital level

ICU is the place of greatest exposure for hospital patients. The most severely ill patients are in ICU and frequently, these patients are more immunosuppressed, so they have more risk of CRBSIs. Although ICU patients are generally exposed to more medical devices and are more severely ill than other hospitalized patients, CRBSIs remain common in hospital wards outside the ICU; this is due the fact that there are more patients admitted outside ICU and preventive measures in ICU are greater than elsewhere.

The hospital level influences in the risk of CRBSI. The first level hospitals have more risk than other hospitals. This is due the fact that first level hospitals have more complex patients, that usually they need long and difficult care [8].

Pathogenesis

CRBSIs can be attributable to four major sources, two of them are common (skin colonization and intraluminal contamination) and the other two are rare (Hematogenous seeding and infusate contamination) [9-10].

- Skin colonization: The most common source of CRBSI is colonization of the intracutaneous and intravascular portions of the

catheter by microorganisms from the patient's skin and the hands of health care workers, especially with short-term intravascular devices. Microorganisms gain access to the catheter wound and migrate along the catheter subcutaneous tract into the fibrin sheath that surrounds intravascular catheters. The deposition of biofilm on the external and internal surface of vascular catheters is thought to play an important role in the colonization process.
- Intraluminal contamination (or hub contamination): It´s an important source of CRBSI in patients with CVCs that are in place for more than two weeks or in patients with a surgically implanted device.
- Hematogenous seeding: It can occur during a bacteremia originating from another focus of infection, often from a gastrointestinal site; this is most likely to occur in critically ill patients or those with long-term catheters.
- Infusate contamination: Administration of contaminated infusate or additives, can result in a CRBSI. Now, it's a rare source of CRBSI and generally causes epidemic infections.

Microbiology

The most common bacteria that produce CRBSI are the same as the patient's skin microbiome, because it is the most frequent pathogenic pathway. Gram-positive aerobes, Candida spp. and gram-negative bacilli are the most frequent bacterial groups, highlighting coagulase negative staphylococci. Polymicrobial infections are infrequently involved (<10%) [11].

Gram-positive aerobes bacteria represent two thirds of the CRBSIs (60-70%). Coagulase negative staphylococci is the most frequent group (specially Staphylococcus epidermidis) followed by Staphylococcus aureus and Enterococcus sp. These bacteria are found in the patient's skin, colonizing the catheter, which can cause CRBSIs. In hemodialysis patients, these organisms are responsible for most CRBSIs, as a result of having a catheter for a long time (reflecting skin microbiome) [12].

Gram-negative bacilli are an important bacterial group related to CRBSI (15-20%). The most commonly isolated organisms include Escherichia coli, Klebsiella pneumoniae, Pseudomonas sp, Enterobacter sp, Serratia sp, and Acinetobacter sp. It should be suspected in burn patients (Pseudomonas sp.) and oncology patients (translocation of gut bacteria in patients with altered mucosal barriers). When multiple cases of CRBSIs with gram-negative bacilli should prompt suspicion of an infusate contamination.

Fungi, specially Candida sp. is the last important group related to CRBSI (15-20%). It should be suspected in patients with parenteral nutrition (high concentration of glucose in intravenous hyperalimentation), in immunosuppressed patients and in patients who have received multiple antibacterial antibiotics (for the resistance).

Clinical

Usually, clinical manifestations of CRBSI are non-specific. Fever, inflammation or purulence at the catheter insertion site, hemodynamic instability, altered mental status and catheter dysfunction are some of clinical manifestations of CRBSI. Fever and abrupt onset of septic physiology are the most common clinical manifestations of CRBSI; however, both are also associated with other causes of infection as well as non-infectious etiologies [13].

Peripheral catheters infections often show local symptoms (inflammation at the catheter insertion site, catheter dysfunction) and central catheters infections show systemic symptoms (Fever, hemodynamic instability, altered mental status). Clinical improvement within 24 hours following catheter removal is suggestive of CRBSI (but not sufficient for definitive Presence of inflammation or purulence at the insertion site has high specificity.

Sometimes, CRBSI can be associated with complications including septic thrombophlebitis, infective endocarditis and metastatic musculoskeletal infection. Clinical manifestations reflecting these complications may be present at the time of initial presentation and/or may develop subsequently. These conditions can occur in the context of CRBSI or independently of CRBSI: [14]

- Septic thrombophlebitis refers to venous thrombosis associated with inflammation in the setting of bacteremia. It should be suspected in patients with CRBSI and persistent bacteremia after 72 hours of appropriate therapy. Clinical manifestations may include fever, erythema, a palpable tender cord, and/or purulent drainage and complications include septic pulmonary emboli and secondary pneumonia.

- Infective endocarditis refers to infection of one or more heart valves. It should be suspected in patients with CRBSI or bacteremia >48 to 72 hours with a pathogen associated with infective endocarditis. When *Staphylococcus aureus, Enterococcus* spp. or *Candida* spp. are diagnosed, echocardiogra-phy is mandatory.
- Metastatic musculoskeletal infection (such as septic arthritis, osteomyelitis and orthopedic hardware infection), the bacteremia may be associated with seeding of joints, bone, or orthopedic hardware. It should be suspected in patients with acute onset musculoskeletal pain.

Diagnosis

The diagnosis of CRBSI is based on clinical factors and laboratory tests, highlighting the cultures, both blood cultures and catheter cultures.

Clinical Factors
CRBSI should be suspected in patients with fever, or hypotension in the setting of a catheter placed at least 48 hours prior to development of symptoms; however, these manifestations aren't specific, may be caused by other infections and non-infectious etiologies.

Physical examination findings of erythema, pain, swelling, or purulence at the insertion site should also raise suspicion for CRBSI. These patients should also be evaluated for signs and symptoms reflecting complications of CRBSI.

Clinical improvement within 24 hours following catheter removal is suggestive of CRBSI (but not sufficient for definitive diagnosis) [13].

Laboratory Test
The most important laboratory tests are the cultures. Blood culture will be the first laboratory test and, if the catheter is removed, catheter culture should be performed. Other laboratory tests like high white blood cell count, C-reactive protein, and procalcitonin are not useful as specific predictors for CRBSI.

If CRBSI is suspected, blood cultures should be obtained, ideally prior to the initiation of antibiotic/antipyretic therapy. For patients who are clinically stable, antibiotic therapy may be deferred while waiting blood culture results. For patients who are clinically unstable, empiric antibiotic therapy should be initiated (after blood cultures have been obtained) [15].

If blood cultures establish the presence of a bloodstream infection (BSI), the patient should be evaluated for alternative sources (pulmonary, abdominal, urinary tract, bone/joint, or skin/soft tissue infection). If no alternative cause for BSI is identified, the diagnosis of CRBSI can be made clinically based on the presence of primary bacteremia and an indwelling catheter.

Table 1. Diagnosis with and without catheter withdrawal

Diagnosis without catheter withdrawal	Criteria for positivity	Comments
Paired quantitative blood cultures	Both sets are positive for the same microorganism and the set obtained through the catheter has ≥3:1 fold-higher colony count than the peripheral culture	Sensitivity 80% Specificity 95% to 99% Labor intensive and expensive
Paired blood cultures for differential time to positivity (DTP)	Both sets are positive for the same microorganism and the set obtained through the catheter becomes positive ≥120 min earlier	Sensitivity: 72% to 96% Specificity: 90% to 95% Less specificity for long-term catheters. The interpretation should take into account adherence to the technical procedure and the type of microorganism.
Endoluminal brushing	>100 CFU. Indicative of CRBSI	Sensitivity: 95% to 100% Specificity: 84% to 89% It may underestimate CRBSI in short-term catheters. Risk of complications
Superficial cultures (semiquantitative cultures of skin surrounding the entry)	≥15 CFU per plate. Indicative of CRBSI	Sensitivity: 78% Specificity: 92% Must be combined with peripheral blood culture
Gram stain-acridine orange leukocyte cytospin of catheter blood	Presence of any microorganisms in a minimum of 100 high-powered fields. Indicative of CRBSI	Sensitivity ≈ 79% Specificity ≈ 87% The technique is simple and rapid, but requires cytospin technology
Semiquantitative catheter culture	≥15 CFU. The same microorganism in at least one percutaneous blood culture and catheter tip culture	Sensitivity ≈ 84% Specificity ≈ 86% It detects colonization on the external surface
Quantitative catheter segment culture	>100 CFU. The same microorganism in at least one percutaneous blood culture and catheter tip culture	Sensitivity ≈ 83% Specificity ≈ 91% All quantitative methods are time consuming
Gram stain-acridine orange leukocyte cytospin	Presence of any microorganisms in a minimum of 100 high-powered fields.	Sensitivity ≈ 85% Specificity ≈ 90% Labor intensive

Ideally, at least two sets of blood cultures should be obtained from peripheral veins via separate venipuncture sites prior to initiation of antibiotic therapy. When this is not possible, one blood culture set can be drawn from a peripheral vein and the other blood culture set can be drawn from the catheter. Blood cultures should not be drawn only from the catheter, since this site may be colonized with skin contaminants, so, at least one blood culture set should be drawn from a peripheral vein. Catheter colonization should be suspected in cases where a single positive culture for skin bacteria (Coagulase negative staphylococci).

The microbiological confirmation diagnosis of CRBSI can be made by microbiological techniques once the catheter has been removed, or before it is removed. Table 1 shows the interpretation of cultures for the diagnosis of CRBSI [16].

Prevention

The best way to avoid and treatment CRBSIs is to prevent them. All intravascular devices confer a risk of infection but, following the prevention guidelines, CRBSIs will decrease significantly, since the best treatment for CRBSIs is prevention.

Strict adherence to hand hygiene recommendations and the use of aseptic techniques during insertion and dressing changes remain the most important measures for the prevention of CRBSI [6, 13].

Other important preventive measures include: choosing appropriate sites for catheter insertion, using the appropriate catheter, using barrier precautions during insertion, ensuring proper catheter site care and removal of catheters when no longer essential. Prevention has three key points: characteristics related to the catheter, site care and catheter care.

Catheter Related
Choosing the most appropriate catheter characteristics for each moment is very important for prevention.

Type of Catheter
As described before, all intravascular devices confer a risk of infection, although some carry greater risk than others. Central arterial catheter is the catheter with the highest risk and PICC is the catheter with lowest risk.

Peripheral venous catheter has low risk infection and CVCs have more risk than peripheral venous catheter, but not all CVCs have the same risk; non-tunneled CVCs have more risk than tunneled CVCs and tunneled CVCs have more risk than totally implantable CVCs.

Anatomic Location

The anatomic site chosen for catheter placement influences the subsequent risk for catheter-associated infection.

In peripheral intravenous catheters, the risk of infection is higher in the lower extremity compared with the upper extremity, and higher in the wrist or upper arm compared with the hand.

In CVCs, the risk of infection is higher in femoral veins than internal jugular veins. Subclavian veins have a lower risk in CVCs [17].

Duration

The duration of catheterization has been considered an important risk factor for infection with both venous and arterial catheters. It is prudent to remove the catheters when no longer needed. Catheters should not be replaced routinely. Usually, when CRBSI is suspected, the best treatment is to remove the catheter, but when central venous catheters are replaced, it's not recommended to use guidewire exchange techniques.

The risk of infection depending on the duration of the catheter changes according to the type of catheter; for peripheral intravenous catheter the risk is greater than three to four days; for CVC the risk is greater than six days and for arterial catheter the risk is greater than four to six days.

If adherence to aseptic technique cannot be assured (emergent catheter placement), it suggests catheter replacement as soon as possible (and no longer than 48 hours after insertion) [18].

Catheter Material

Peripheral intravenous catheters composed of Teflon or polyurethane have fewer complications. For central catheter, a number of catheter materials have been evaluated to minimize the risk of infection (Chlorhexidine-silver sulfadiazine-impregnated catheters, silver-impregnated collagen cuff catheters, heparin-bonded catheters) It suggests use of antimicrobial-impregnated catheters

Site Care

It's important to use an antiseptic solution (chlorhexidine) for skin disinfection at the catheter insertion site reduces the risk of infection. It's also important for the sterile technique for minimizing CRBSI. This includes strict adherence to hand washing and aseptic technique and, with central venous catheter (CVC) insertion, sterile gloves, long-sleeved surgical gown, a surgical mask, and a large sterile sheet drape.

The type of dressing at the insertion site may affect the rate of catheter infection. Sterile gauze or sterile, transparent, semipermeable dressing should be used to cover the catheter site. If the patient is diaphoretic or if the site is bleeding or oozing, a gauze dressing should be used. The catheter site dressing should be replaced if the dressing becomes damp or soiled.

It is not recommended to use topical antibiotic ointment or cream on the insertion site except dialysis catheters because increased rates of antimicrobial resistance [13]

Catheter Care

It's important for access point management; contaminated needleless connectors, catheter hubs, or injection ports are causes for CRBSI. It recommends wiping the access port with an appropriate antiseptic and accessing the port only with sterile devices to avoid risk catheter infection.

Studies suggest the use of heparin-bonded CVCs in patients with hematologic or oncologic malignancy reduce risk catheter infection (reduce risk thrombosis) but, in general, it's not recommended routine use of anticoagulation to reduce the risk of catheter-related infection.

Antibiotic locks are not recommended routine use except for patients with long-term catheters (especially hemodialysis) and a history of recurrent CRBSI despite adherence to other routine infection prevention measures [6].

Treatment

In general, management of CRBSI consists of catheter removal (if feasible) and systemic antibiotic therapy, but there are special conditions that can change the usual treatment, especially in hemodialysis patients.

When CRBSI is suspected, the patient should be evaluated, start empirical antibiotic treatment and decide whether to remove or salvage the catheter.

When the infection has produced a peripheral catheter, treatment consists of removing the catheter. Conversely, for central catheter (specially CVCs), patient evaluation is the key to deciding whether to remove or salvage the catheter, although, as far as possible, the recommendation is to remove it.

The catheter must be removed when one of the conditions is associated:

- Sepsis or hemodynamic instability
- Presence of concomitant endocarditis or evidence of metastatic infection
- Presence of suppurative thrombophlebitis
- Presence of a propagating clot
- Persistent bacteremia after 72 hours of appropriate antimicrobial therapy
- Subcutaneously tunneled central venous catheter tunnel tract infection or subcutaneous port reservoir infection
- It suggests to remove catheter when the infection is suspected due to *S. aureus*, *P. aeruginosa*, drug-resistant gram-negative bacilli, *Enterococcus* spp or *Candida* spp. Catheter must be removed when CRBSI is confirmed for these pathogens [16].

Catheter salvage or guidewire exchange may be considered if catheter removal is not feasible (there is no alternative access site or access sites are limited, the patient has a bleeding diathesis, the patient declines removal, or quality of life issues take priority over the need for catheter reinsertion at another site). Catheter salvage should not be attempted in patients with a condition warranting catheter removal.

The combination of a glycopeptide (vancomycin at doses of 15 mg/kg every 12 hours if renal function is normal) or daptomycin at doses not less than 6mg/kg every 24 h), associated with a third generation cephalosporin (ceftriaxone 2gr IV every 24 hours) or **aminoglycoside** (amikacin at doses conventional daily only) is empirical antibiotic treatment.

If *P. aeruginosa* is suspected (In patients with neutropenia or severe burns) antipseudomonal antibiotics should be added (piperacillin-tazobactam 4gr every 8h, ceftazidime 2gr every 8h). If multiresistant gram-negative bacteria are suspected, empirical coverage with a carbapenem (imipenem or meropenem at the usual doses) should be evaluated.

Echinocandins are currently recommended for empirical therapy if *Candida* spp. is suspected in patients with severe infections. Fluconazole (800 mg loading dose, then 400 mg daily) is the initial treatment although it can use anidulafungin or amphotericin B.

Table 2. Specific treatment for CRBSI

Pathogen	Preferred antibiotics	Alternative antibiotics
Staphylococci		
Methicillin susceptible	Cefazolin 2gr IV/8h	Vancomycin (same dose)
Methicillin resistant	Vancomycin: Loading dose: 20-35mg/kg IV Maintenance dose and interval: determined by nomogram; usually 15-20 mg/kg IV/8-12 h	Daptomycin 6-10mg/kg IV/24h
Enterococci		
Ampicillin susceptible	Ampicillin 2gr IV/4h	Vancomycin (same dose)
Ampicillin resistant	Vancomycin (same dose)	Daptomycin (same dose) Linezolid 600mg IV/12h
Enterobacteriaceae		
Extended-spectrum beta-lactamase negative	Ceftriaxone 2gr IV/24h	Ciprofloxacin 400mg IV/12h
Extended-spectrum beta-lactamase positive	- Imipenem 500mg IV/6h - Meropenem 1gr IV/8h - Ertapenem 1gr IV/24h	Ciprofloxacin (same dose)
Pseudomonas spp.	- Ceftazidime 2gr IV/8h - Cefepime 2gr IV/8h - Piperacillin-tazobactam 4.5gr IV/6h	Imipenem (same dose) Meropenem (same dose) Ciprofloxacin (same dose)
Candida spp.	Fluconazole: Loading dose: 800mg IV Maintenance: 400mg IV/24h	Anidulafungin: Loading dose: 200mg IV Maintenance 100mg IV/24h

Antibiotic lock therapy (ALT) provides a concentrated antibiotic solution into the catheter lumen to achieve a drug level high enough to kill bacteria within the biofilm of the catheter. Anticoagulants are thought to be beneficial in ALT for treatment of CRBSI by interfering with fibrin formation and allowing increased antibiotic penetration into microbial biofilm. In general, ALT is used as adjunctive therapy together with systemic antibiotics for treatment CRBSI in the setting of catheter salvage; It includes patients with a long-term intravascular device (hemodialysis, parenteral nutrition) who are hemodynamically stable with CRBSI due to a pathogen of relatively low virulence in the absence of complications. The most commonly used antibiotics are vancomycin, cefazolin, ceftazidime and gentamicin. Potential adverse effects of ALT include systemic toxicity, antibiotic resistance and secondary candidemia. Usually, ALT should be maintained between 14-28 days [19].

The antibiotic treatment time changes depending on whether the catheter is saved or removed. When the catheter is removed, the duration of treatment is 7 to 14 days. When the catheter is saved, the duration of treatment is 14 to 21 days.

Once the pathogen is confirmed, the empirical treatment should be modified. The specific treatment of each pathogen is shown in Table 2 [16, 19].

Conclusion

Currently, it´s estimated that catheter-related bloodstream infections are responsible for between 15% and 30% of nosocomial bacteremia. All intravascular devices confer a risk of infection, although it´s estimated that between 75-90% of CRBSIs occur with Central Venous Catheters. Gram-positive aerobes bacteria represent two thirds of the CRBSIs (60-70%). Strict adherence to hand hygiene recommendations and the use of aseptic techniques during insertion and dressing changes remain the most important measures for the prevention of CRBSI. In general, management of CRBSIs consist of catheter removal (if feasible) and systemic antibiotic therapy.

References

[1] Mermel LA. Short-term Peripheral Venous Catheter-Related Bloodstream Infections: A Systematic Review. *Clin Infect Dis* 2017; 65:1757.

[2] Ferrer C, Almirante B. Infecciones relacionadas con el uso de los catéteres vasculares [Venous catheter-related infections]. *Enferm Infecc Microbiol Clin.* 2014;32(2):115-124.

[3] Beekmann SE, Henderson DK. Infections caused by percutaneous intravascular devices. En: Mandell GL, Bennett JE, Dolin R, editores. *Mandell, Douglas and Bennett's Principles and Practice of Infectious Diseases.* Philadelphia: Churchill Livingstone - Elsevier; 2010. p. 3697–715.

[4] Centers for Disease Control and Prevention (CDC). Vital signs: central line-associated blood stream infections--United States, 2001, 2008, and 2009. *MMWR Morb Mortal Wkly Rep* 2011; 60:243.

[5] Reunes S, Rombaut V, Vogelaers D, et al. Risk factors and mortality for nosocomial bloodstream infections in elderly patients. *Eur J Intern Med* 2011; 22:e39.

[6] Maki DG, Kluger DM, Crnich CJ. The risk of bloodstream infection in adults with different intravascular devices: a systematic review of 200 published prospective studies. *Mayo Clin Proc* 2006; 81:1159.

[7] Parienti JJ, du Cheyron D, Timsit JF, et al. Meta-analysis of subclavian insertion and nontunneled central venous catheter-associated infection risk reduction in critically ill adults. *Crit Care Med* 2012; 40:1627.

[8] Coello R, Charlett A, Ward V, Wilson J, Pearson A, Sedgwick J, et al. Device Related sources of bacteraemia in English hospitals - opportunities for the prevention of hospital-acquired bacteraemia. *J Hosp Infect.* 2003;53:46–57.

[9] Pascual A. Pathogenesis of catheter-related infections: Lessons for new designs. *Clin Microbiol Infect.* 2002;8:256–64.

[10] Liñares J, Sitges-Serra A, Garau J, Pérez JL, Martín R. Pathogenesis of catheter sepsis: A prospective study with quantitative and semiquantitative cultures of catheter hub and segments. *J Clin Microbiol.* 1985;21:357–60.

[11] Maki DG. Nosocomial bacteremia. An epidemiologic overview. *Am J Med* 1981; 70:719.

[12] Weiner LM, Webb AK, Limbago B, et al. Antimicrobial-Resistant Pathogens Associated With Healthcare-Associated Infections: Summary of Data Reported to the National Healthcare Safety Network at the Centers for Disease Control and Prevention, 2011-2014. *Infect Control Hosp Epidemiol* 2016; 37:1288.

[13] O'Grady NP, Barie PS, Bartlett JG, et al. Guidelines for evaluation of new fever in critically ill adult patients: 2008 update from the American College of Critical Care Medicine and the Infectious Diseases Society of America. *Crit Care Med* 2008; 36:1330.

[14] Farrington CA, Allon M. Complications of Hemodialysis Catheter Bloodstream Infections: Impact of Infecting Organism. *Am J Nephrol* 2019; 50:126.

[15] Miller JM, Binnicker MJ, Campbell S, et al. A Guide to Utilization of the Microbiology Laboratory for Diagnosis of Infectious Diseases: 2018 Update by the Infectious Diseases Society of America and the American Society for Microbiology. *Clin Infect Dis* 2018; 67:e1.

[16] Chaves F, Garnacho-Montero J, Del Pozo JL, et al. Diagnosis and treatment of catheter-related bloodstream infection: Clinical guidelines of the Spanish Society of Infectious Diseases and Clinical Microbiology and (SEIMC) and the Spanish Society of Spanish Society of Intensive and Critical Care Medicine and Coronary Units (SEMICYUC). *Med Intensiva.* 2018;42(1):5-36.

[17] Parienti JJ, Mongardon N, Mégarbane B, et al. Intravascular Complications of Central Venous Catheterization by Insertion Site. *N Engl J Med* 2015; 373:1220.
[18] Webster J, Osborne S, Rickard CM, Marsh N. Clinically-indicated replacement versus routine replacement of peripheral venous catheters. *Cochrane Database Syst Rev* 2019; 1:CD007798.
[19] Mermel LA, Allon M, Bouza E, et al. Clinical practice guidelines for the diagnosis and management of intravascular catheter-related infection: 2009 Update by the Infectious Diseases Society of America. *Clin Infect Dis* 2009; 49:1.

Chapter 8

Endocarditis and Intravascular Infections

Covadonga Martín Garrido*, RN
Department of Nursery, Hospital del Tajo, Madrid, Spain

Abstract

In this chapter we are going to break down infective endocarditis, knowing its pathology, etiology and treatment.

Keywords: infective endocarditis (IE), prevention, treatment, intravascular infections

Introduction

Infective endocarditis (IE) is the proliferation of microorganisms in the cardiac endothelium. The characteristic lesion of endocarditis at the site of infection is vegetation, which consists of a mass of platelets, inflammatory cells, and microorganisms. Endocarditis most frequently affects heart valves (native or prosthetic), but it also affects areas of mural endocardium damaged by blood jets or some foreign bodies such as implantable devices (pacemakers or defibrillators) or intravascular catheters [1].

In developed countries, the incidence of IE varies between 1.5 and 6.2 cases per 100,000 inhabitants per year. The incidence of IE is markedly

---

* Corresponding Author's E-mail: Covadonga1995_MG@hotmail.com.

In: Nosocomial Infection in Abdominal Surgery
Editors: Jaime Ruiz-Tovar and Andrés García Marín
ISBN: 978-1-68507-603-0
© 2022 Nova Science Publishers, Inc.

increased in the elderly and in parenteral drug addicts. The cumulative rate of IE of prosthetic valves is 1.5 to 3.0% one year after valve replacement and 3 to 6% at five years; the risk of IE is highest during the first six months after valve replacement. Despite improvements in its management, IE continues to be associated with high mortality and severe complications [1]. The in-hospital mortality rate of patients with IE varies from 15 to 30% [2].

Etiology

IE can be caused by various types of microorganisms, including multiple species of bacteria and fungi. However, most cases are due to a small number of bacterial species. The causative microorganisms vary among the different clinical types of endocarditis, in part because of their different portals of entry [2].

Prevention of Endocarditis

Antibiotic prophylaxis is considered indicated to prevent IE, only to high-risk patients (patients with the highest incidence of IE or highest risk of adverse clinical outcomes resulting from IE), and only in certain procedures [3, 4].

High-risk patients:

1. Patients with a prosthetic valve or prosthetic material used for valvuloplasty, transcatheter valve prostheses, and allografts.
2. Patients with previous IE
3. Patients with untreated cyanotic congenital heart disease (CHD) and those with CHD with palliative postoperative shunts, conduits or other prostheses [4].

Antibiotic prophylaxis is not indicated for other types of valvulopathy or congenital heart disease [3].

Risk procedures: Dental procedures requiring manipulation of the gingival or periapical region of the tooth or perforation of the oral mucosa [3].

IE prophylaxis is not indicated for all other procedures: respiratory, gastrointestinal or genitourinary tract procedures, including vaginal or cesarean delivery, or dermatological or musculoskeletal procedures [3].

Aseptic measures are mandatory during insertion and manipulation of venous catheters and during invasive procedures, including outpatient procedures, to reduce the rate of IE associated with diagnostic and therapeutic procedures. Antibiotic treatment is only necessary when invasive procedures are performed in the context of infection [3].

Recommended prophylaxis for high-risk dental procedures in high-risk patients: Amoxicillin or Ampicillin 2 g oral or IV, single dose 30-60 min before the procedure (in allergic patients: Clindamycin 600 mg, oral or IV) [5].

Prophylaxis in cardiac and/or vascular interventions: Perioperative antibiotic prophylaxis should be considered for patients undergoing prosthetic valve implantation (surgical or transcatheter), any type of prosthetic graft or pacemaker, due to the increased risk of infection and adverse outcome [3]. The organisms that most frequently cause early prosthetic valve infections (1 year after surgery) are coagulase-negative staphylococci (CNS) and *Staphylococcus aureus*. Prophylaxis should be started immediately before the procedure, repeated if the procedure is long and completed 48 h later. Preoperative screening for nasal S. aureus carriers is recommended before elective cardiac surgery to treat carriers with mupirocin and local chlorhexidine [4].

Diagnosis of IE

Clinical History

The clinical history of IE is extremely variable depending on the causative organism, the presence or absence of pre-existing heart disease, the presence or absence of prosthetic valves or cardiac devices, and the form of presentation [1].

The most frequent symptoms are fever (90%), chills, anorexia, weight loss, heart murmurs (85%) and embolic phenomena (25%) [1].

Laboratory

Patients with IE often have laboratory data indicative of infection, such as elevated C-reactive protein (CRP), erythrocyte sedimentation rate (ESR), leukocytosis, anemia, and microscopic hematuria, although these signs lack specificity [1].

Imaging Diagnosis of IE

Echocardiography: Transthoracic echocardiography (TTE) is the technique of choice for the diagnosis of IE and plays an essential role in the management and monitoring of these patients [5]. Echocardiography should be performed as soon as IE is suspected. Transesophageal echocardiography (TEE) should be performed when there is a high index of suspicion of IE, especially if TTE is of suboptimal quality and to rule out complications [5].

The echocardiographic findings considered the main diagnostic criteria for IE are vegetation, abscess or pseudoaneurysm, and new dehiscence of a valve prosthesis. The sensitivity of TTE for the diagnosis of vegetations in native and prosthetic valves is 70% and 50%, respectively, and that of TEE is 96% and 92%. The specificity described for both TTE and TEE is around 90% [5].

Multislice CT: useful for detecting abscesses and pseudoaneurysms with a diagnostic accuracy similar to that of TEE, as well as for assessing perivalvular extension, including the anatomy of pseudoaneurysm, abscesses and fistulas. It can also be useful for the diagnosis of embolic complications (although MRI is more sensitive in these cases) [5, 11].

MRI: used to detect embolic complications of IE (cerebral, splenic) [5].

Nuclear cardiology imaging techniques: molecular nuclear techniques (SPECT/CT and (18) F-FDG/CT) are a supplementary method in patients with suspected IE and diagnostic difficulties [5, 11].

Microbiological Diagnosis of IE

Positive blood cultures remain the cornerstone of IE diagnosis and provide live bacteria for both identification and antibiotic susceptibility testing. At least three blood samples should be taken at 30 min intervals, each of 10 ml volume. The blood culture must be obtained before antibiotic administration. In IE, bacteremia is constant, so there is no reason to delay blood sampling when there are fever peaks; virtually all blood cultures are positive [2].

IE with negative blood culture (occurs in 30%) usually appears as a consequence of previous antibiotic treatment, so it is necessary to withdraw antibiotic therapy and repeat the blood culture [2].

Histological Diagnosis

Pathological examination of resected valve tissue or embolic fragments remains the gold standard for the diagnosis of IE [1].

Diagnostic Criteria for Endocarditis

In the latest 2015 European Society of Cardiology endocarditis guidelines, new IE criteria have been defined, where value is added to imaging tests [1].

Prognosis of IE

The in-hospital mortality rate for patients with IE ranges from 15-30%. Rapid identification of patients at increased risk of death may be an opportunity to change the course of the disease (i.e., emergency or urgent surgery) and improve diagnosis. The prognosis of IE is influenced by four main factors: patient characteristics, the presence or absence of cardiac and noncardiac complications, the infectious organism, and echocardiographic findings [2].

Treatment

Empirical Treatment

Treatment of IE should be initiated immediately. Three sets of blood cultures should be drawn at 30 min intervals before starting antibiotic therapy [6].
    Antibiotic regimens for community-acquired IE should cover staphylococci, streptococci and enterococococci: administer Ampicillin 12 g/day i.v. in 4-6 doses + cloxacillin or oxacillin 12 g/day i. v. in 4-6 doses + Gentamicin 3 mg/kg/day i.v. or i.m. in 1 dose (for penicillin-allergic patients: Vancomycin 30-60 mg/kg/day i.v. in 2-3 doses + Gentamicin 3 mg/kg/day i.v. or i.m. in 1 dose) [6].

Regimens for IE in early valve prostheses or IE associated with diagnostic and therapeutic procedures should cover methicillin-resistant staphylococci, enterococci and, ideally, non-HACEK Gram-negative pathogens: administer Vancomycin 30 mg/kg/day i.v. in 2 doses + Gentamicin 3 mg/kg/day i.v. or i.m. in 1 dose + Rifampicin 900-1,200 mg i.v. or orally divided in 2 or 3 doses [6].

Once the pathogen is identified (usually in less than 48 h), antibiotic treatment should be adapted to the microbial sensitivity pattern [6].

Antimicrobial Therapy

Successful treatment of IE is based on the suppression of microbes with antimicrobial drugs [6].

Surgical Treatment

Approximately half of the patients with IE require surgical treatment due to severe complications [8]. Surgery contributes by removing infected material and allowing abscesses to drain [7].

The three main indications for early surgery in IE are heart failure, uncontrolled infection and prevention of embolic complications [7]. Cardiac surgery in IE is indicated if:

IE causes severe valvular insufficiency or obstruction causing symptoms of HF or with echocardiographic signs of poor hemodynamic tolerance.

Infection is locally uncontrolled (abscess, pseudoaneurysm, fistula, growing vegetation).

Persistently positive blood cultures despite adequate antibiotic treatment and control of septic metastatic foci.

IE of prosthetic valve caused by staphylococci or non-HACEK Gram-negative bacteria.

IE caused by fungi or multidrug-resistant microorganisms.

Persistent vegetations >10 mm after at least 1 embolic episode despite adequate antibiotic treatment [7, 12].

Intravascular Infections

Intravascular infections are very common; in the United States, approximately 80,000 central venous catheter infections occur in intensive care units each year [9].

Infection, phlebitis and less frequently, bacteremia are common problems associated with intravascular catheters inserted in patients during hospital admission. Most serious infections are associated with central venous catheters (CVC) in patients admitted to the ICU [13, 15].

The prevention of intravascular infections involves proper aseptic puncture technique and hand hygiene [16]. Other prevention measures are: choosing the right site and material for puncture and removing catheters when they are not essential [10, 15].

Three risk factors for intravascular catheter infection have been identified: the type, location and duration of the inserted catheter. All catheters are associated with a risk of infection, although peripheral lines have a lower risk of infection than central catheters; of these, the femoral venous line has a higher risk than the jugular or subclavian line. The risk of infection increases with the duration of catheterization, increasing when it is inserted for more than 3 to 6 days (it is advisable not to keep peripheral lines for more than 7 days; if the line has been inserted in an emergency situation, it is recommended to change it after 48 hours) [15, 18].

The puncture site of the intravascular catheter should be monitored daily; its removal is indicated if signs of infection are detected [15].

The use of intravascular catheters impregnated with antimicrobial or antiseptic substances (chlorhexidine, sulfadiazine, minocycline-rifampin) has been shown to reduce the incidence of intravascular infections in patients admitted to the ICU [15].

Other preventive measures to minimize intravascular infections are:

1. Adequate hand hygiene with alcoholic solutions or soap with antiseptics (the use of gloves does not supersede adequate hand hygiene).
2. Catheter insertion procedure with sterile gloves and gown, surgical mask, sterile drapes.
3. Skin disinfection with chlorhexidine-alcohol (air dry before puncture).
4. Avoid femoral puncture.

5. Remove catheters when there is no indication.
6. Antibiotic creams on the puncture site are not indicated (they might promote resistance and fungal colonization) [14, 15].

In general, the diagnosis of intravascular infections is reached by an adequate clinical evaluation and microbiological confirmation with blood cultures obtained from the catheter or from a peripheral vein [15, 18].

Intravascular infection with bacteremia should always be suspected when there is a febrile condition in a patient with a central venous catheter and no other apparent source of infection. Fever (>38°) is the main symptom. Other clinical manifestations include hemodynamic instability, altered mental status, catheter dysfunction or clinical signs of sudden onset sepsis after catheter insertion. Clinical improvement 24 hours after catheter removal is suggestive of intravascular infection [10, 15].

Positive blood cultures for species such as S. aureus, coagulase-negative staphylococci, or Candida in the absence of other sources of infection should raise suspicion of intravascular infection. Catheter and peripheral vein cultures should be obtained before starting antibiotic treatment. The same microorganism should be obtained in the catheter and peripheral blood cultures (at least two blood cultures) [17].

The treatment of intravascular infections requires removal of the infected catheter (exceptionally, conservative management of bacteremia by sealing the vascular catheters with antimicrobials) and antibiotic treatment [18].

Treatment is influenced by a number of important factors: the type of device and its method of insertion, the pathogen causing the infection, the existence of associated immunosuppression or neutropenia, the presence of comorbidities or other prosthetic materials (especially cardiovascular or orthopedic), the possibility of obtaining alternative venous access, the expected duration of vascular catheterization, and the nature and severity of the infection itself [1, 2].

Non-permanent catheters should be removed whenever they are suspected to be the source of bacteremia; they should also be removed if they have local signs of infection, even if there is no bacteremia. Indwelling catheters should also be removed if there is bacteremia; the risk of not removing a catheter that is causing an infection is to provoke recurrent bacteremia and possible metastatic infections. The replacement of a CVC originating an infection, by means of a guidewire system, has a high risk of recurrence and possible embolization, so its routine practice is contraindicated [18].

Empirical antibiotic treatment should be started, which should include antimicrobials active against gram-positive and gram-negative microorganisms that most often cause these infections. In general, vancomycin should be administered at a dose of 15 mg/kg every 12 h (another option is daptomycin at a dose of not less than 6 mg/kg every 24 h). Subsequently, the antibiotic should be guided according to the result of the antibiogram [18].

Treatment according to the germ:

- *S. aureus*, if sensitive to methicillin: cloxacillin (at a dose of 2 g every 4 h) or cefazolin (at a dose of 1-2 g every 8 h). In infections caused by MRSA or if there is allergy to beta-lactams: vancomycin, daptomycin or linezolid.
- Gram-negative bacilli: cephalosporins, monobactams, carbapenems or fluorinated quinolones.
- *Candida* species: fluconazole (400 to 800 mg per day) [6].

The duration of therapy should be 10 to 14 days (day 1 is considered the first day that blood cultures are negative). Patients with persistent bacteremia >72 hours after catheter removal should be studied to rule out complications of intravascular infection such as suppurative thrombophlebitis, endocarditis or metastatic foci of infection (in these cases, they should receive antibiotic treatment for at least 6 weeks) [6].

Antibiotic treatment is not indicated if:

- Positive catheter culture, in the absence of signs of infection.
- Positive blood cultures obtained through the catheter with negative blood cultures obtained through a peripheral vein.
- Signs of phlebitis in the absence of infection [6, 9].

Conclusion

Infective endocarditis (IE) is the proliferation of microorganisms in the cardiac endothelium. Despite improvements in its management, IE continues to be associated with high mortality and severe complications. Antibiotic prophylaxis is considered indicated to prevent IE, only to high-risk patients

(patients with the highest incidence of IE or highest risk of adverse clinical outcomes resulting from IE), and only in certain procedures.

Infection, phlebitis and less frequently, bacteremia are common problems associated with intravascular catheters inserted in patients during hospital admission. Most serious infections are associated with central venous catheters (CVC) in patients admitted to the ICU. Intravascular infection may lead to bacteremia and sepsis. The best method for prevention of intravascular infection is the aseptic insertion of the catheter. The puncture site of the intravascular catheter should be monitored daily; its removal is indicated if signs of infection are detected.

References

[1] Thuny F, Grisoli D, Collart F, Habib G, Raoult D. Management of infective endocarditis: challenges and perspectives. *Lancet.* 2012;379:965-75.
[2] Leone S, Ravasio V, Durante-Mangoni E, Crapis M, Carosi G, Scotton PG, Barzaghi N, Falcone M, Chinello P, Pasticci MB, Grossi P, Utili R, Viale P, Rizzi M, Suter F. Epidemiology, characteristics, and outcome of infective endocarditis in Italy: the Italian Study on *Endocarditis. Infection.* 2012;40:527-35.
[3] De Oliveira JC, Martinelli M, Nishioka SA, Varejao T, Uipe D, Pedrosa AA, Costa R, D'Avila A, Danik SB. Efficacy of antibiotic prophylaxis before the implantation of pacemakers and cardioverter-defibrillators: results of a large, prospective, randomized, double-blinded, placebo-controlled trial. *Circ. Arrhythm. Electrophysiol.* 2009;2:29-34.
[4] Bode LG, Kluytmans JA, Wertheim HF, Bogaers D, Vandenbroucke-Grauls CM, Roosendaal R, Troelstra A, Box AT, Voss A, van der Tweel I, van Belkum A, Verbrugh HA, Vos MC. Preventing surgical-site infections in nasal carriers of Staphylococcus aureus. *N Engl. J. Med.* 2010;362:9-17.
[5] Habib G, Badano L, Tribouilloy C, Vilacosta I, Zamorano JL, Galderisi M, Voigt JU, Sicari R, Cosyns B, Fox K, Aakhus S. Recommendations for the practice of echocardiography in infective endocarditis. *Eur. J. Echocardiogr.* 2010;11:202-19.
[6] 2015 ESC Guidelines for the management of infective endocarditis: The Task Force for the Management of Infective Endocarditis of the European Society of Cardiology (ESC) *Eur. Heart J.* 2015; 36 (44): 3075-3128.
[7] Thuny F, Beurtheret S, Mancini J, Gariboldi V, Casalta JP, Riberi A, Giorgi R, Gouriet F, Tafanelli L, Avierinos JF, Renard S, Collart F, Raoult D, Habib G. The timing of surgery influences mortality and morbidity in adults

with severe complicated infective endocarditis: a propensity analysis. *Eur. Heart J.* 2011;32:2027-33.

[8] Vahanian A, Alfieri O, Andreotti F, Antunes MJ, Baron-Esquivias G, Baumgartner H, Borger MA, Carrel TP, De Bonis M, Evangelista A, Falk V, Iung B, Lancellotti P, Pierard L, Price S, Schafers HJ, Schuler G, Stepinska J, Swedberg K, Takkenberg J, von Oppell UO, Windecker S, Zamorano JL, Zembala M. Guidelines on the management of valvular heart disease (version 2012). *Eur. Heart J.* 2012;33: 2451-96.

[9] Eggimann P, Waldvogel F. Pacemaker and defibrillator infections. In: *Infections Associated with Indwelling Medical Devices*, Waldvogel FA, Bisno AL (Eds), American Society for Microbiology Press, Washington, DC 2000. p. 247.

[10] Polyzos KA, Konstantelias AA, Falagas ME. Risk factors for cardiac implantable electronic device infection: a systematic review and meta-analysis. *Europace* 2015; 17:767.

[11] Ploux S, Riviere A, Amraoui S, Whinnett Z, Barandon L, Lafitte S, Ritter P, Papaioannou G, Clementy J, Jais P, Bordenave L, Haissaguerre M, Bordachar P. Positron emission tomography in patients with suspected pacing system infections may play a critical role in difficult cases. *Heart Rhythm*. 2011;8: 1478-81.

[12] Sohail MR, Uslan DZ, Khan AH, Friedman PA, Hayes DL, Wilson WR, Steckelberg JM, Jenkins SM, Baddour LM. Infective endocarditis complicating permanent pacemaker and implantable cardioverter-defibrillator infection. *Mayo Clin. Proc.* 2008;83:46-53.

[13] Baddour LM, Epstein AE, Erickson CC, Knight BP, Levison ME, Lockhart PB, Masoudi FA, Okum EJ, Wilson WR, Beerman LB, Bolger AF, Estes NA III, Gewitz M, Newburger JW, Schron EB, Taubert KA. Update on cardiovascular implantable electronic device infections and their management: a scientific statement from the American Heart Association. *Circulation*. 2010;121:458-77.

[14] Grammes JA, Schulze CM, Al Bataineh M, Yesenosky GA, Saari CS, Vrabel MJ, Horrow J, Chowdhury M, Fontaine JM, Kutalek SP. Percutaneous pacemaker and implantable cardioverter-defibrillator lead extraction in 100 patients with intracardiac vegetations defined by transesophageal echocardiogram. *J. Am. Coll. Cardiol.* 2010;55:886-94.

[15] Mermel LA, Allon M, Bouza E, et al. Clinical practice guidelines for the diagnosis and management of intravascular catheter-related infection: 2009 Update by the Infectious Diseases Society of America. *Clin. Infect. Dis.* 2009; 49:1.

[16] Pronovost P, Needham D, Berenholtz S, et al. An intervention to decrease catheter-related bloodstream infections in the ICU. *N. Engl. J. Med.* 2006; 355:2725-2732.
[17] Line-Associated Bloodstream Infection). www.cdc.gov/nhsn/PDFs/pscManual/4PSC_CLABScurrent.pdf (Accessed on April 21, 2021).
[18] Lebeaux D, Fernández-Hidalgo N, Chauhan A, Lee S, Ghigo JM, Almirante B, et al. Management of infections related to totally implantable venous-access ports: Challenges and perspectives. *Lancet Infect. Dis.* 2013; 4: S1473.

Chapter 9

Pseudomembranous Colitis and Other Infections Related to Antibiotics

José Ruiz Pardo[1,*] and Clara Eugenia Cobo Cervantes[2]

[1]Department of General and Digestive Surgery,
Hospital Universitario Torrecárdenas, Almería, Spain
[2]Department of Orthopaedic Surgery and Traumatology,
Hospital Universitario Torrecárdenas, Almería, Spain

Abstract

The chapter summarizes the recent evidence about the management of the pseudomembranous colitis. Moreover, other aspects such as epidemiology, economic impact, pathogenesis, risk factors, clinical features, diagnosis, severity criteria, treatment, infection control and prevention are analyzed.

Keywords: infection, nosocomial infection, pseudomembranous colitis, clostridium difficile

---

[*] Corresponding Author's E-mail: josrp@hotmail.es.

In: Nosocomial Infection in Abdominal Surgery
Editors: Jaime Ruiz-Tovar and Andrés García Marín
ISBN: 978-1-68507-603-0
© 2022 Nova Science Publishers, Inc.

Introduction

Clostridium difficile (C. difficile) is a spore-forming, anaerobic and Gram-positive Bacillus [1], that causes antibiotics-associated diarrhea and pseudomembranous colitis [2]. In Europe, 80% of cases of C. *difficile* infection (CDI) are acquired in hospitalized patients, 14% in the community and 6% are of indeterminate origin [1].

Antibiotics-associated diarrhea affects 5-39% of people treated with antibiotics [3] and it is estimated that *C. difficile* is implicated in 10-25% of cases [4]. In turn, it is calculated that 75% of antibiotic-associated colitis cases are caused by C. *difficile*, and of those, 90-100% are pseudomembranous colitis [5].

Current Evidence

Epidemiology

The incidence of CDI has increased markedly worldwide over the past two decades [4]. Likewise, *C. difficile* is the leading cause of infectious nosocomial diarrhea in developed countries, with a mean incidence of nosocomial cases of 4.1 cases per 10000 patient-days in Europe [1].

Economic Impact

Annual costs for management of CDI amount to approximately $800 million in the USA and €3000 million in Europe. Moreover, estimates suggest that costs associated with recurrent CDI can exceed those of primary CDI [1].

Pathogenesis

CDI is triggered by toxin production from the bacteria. Normal bacterial flora is disrupted, the colon is colonized with the *C. difficile* bacteria, and toxins are released that cause mucosal damage and inflammation. Normal bacterial flora is typically disrupted by antibiotic treatment. The disease can be triggered by nearly any antibiotic, but a study by Slimings and Riley ranked cephalosporins, clindamycin, carbapenems, trimethoprim/sulphonamides, fluoroquinolones and penicillin combinations as the most frequent offenders [6].

C. difficile infection is mediated by two toxins, *C. difficile* toxin A (TcdA) and *C. difficile* toxin B (TcdB), which disrupt tight junctions and destroy the actin cytoskeleton of enterocytes. The toxins induce an inflammatory response by recruiting neutrophils and mastocytes, which release cytokines, leading to the formation of pseudomembranes. Not all patients colonized with *C. difficile* develop CDI. This suggests that other factors such as immune response and intestinal microbiota balance are important in disease pathogenesis [4].

Both the toxins are potent monoglucosyltransferases, active on small GTP-binding proteins (Rho, Rac and Cdc42) involved either in the regulation or in the formation of the cytoskeletal actin in the intestinal epithelium. In addition, some *C. difficile* strains produce a third toxin (binary toxin, CDT), composed of an enzymatic component (CDTa) and a binding component (CDTb). CDTb binds to a cell receptor leading to the internalization of CDTa into the cytosol catalysing the ADP-ribosylation of momomeric actin and the resultant disruption of the actin cytoskeletal [7].

Risk Factors for CDI

Risk factors associated with CDI are described below [6]:

- Antibiotics: cephalosporins, clindamycin, carbapenems, trimethoprim/sulphonamides, fluoroquinolones and penicillin combinations.
- Acid-suppressant medications: proton-pump inhibitors (PPI) especially and H2-receptor antagonists.
- Age >65 years.
- Recent hospitalisation, prolonged hospitalisation (>7 days) or prolonged antibiotic courses.
- Being admitted to a room where the previous patient had CDI.
- Immunosuppression.

Clinical Features

The signs and symptoms of CDI range from self-limited diarrhea to a combination of symptoms which may include fever, elevated white blood cell (WBC) count, abdominal pain and/or distention, and tachycardia. With worsening disease, patients may progress to renal failure, shock, intensive care unit admission, and an acute surgical abdomen [6]. The disease can be classified according to severity into several subtypes [8]:

Mild Disease
Diarrhea as the only symptom.

Moderate Disease
Diarrhea plus any additional signs or symptoms not meeting severe or complicated criteria.

Severe Disease
Serum albumin < 3 g/dl plus ONE of the following:

- WBC count $\geq$ 15,000 cells/mm^3.
- Abdominal tenderness.

Severe and Complicated Disease
Any of the following attributable to CDI:

- Admission to intensive care unit for CDI.
- Hypotension with or without required use of vasopressors.
- Fever $\geq$ 38.5°C.
- Ileus or significant abdominal distention.
- Mental status changes.
- WBC $\geq$ 35,000 cells/mm^3 or < 2,000 cells/mm^3.
- Serum lactate levels > 2.2 mmol/l.
- End organ failure (mechanical ventilation, renal failure, etc…).

Recurrent CDI
Recurrent CDI within 8 weeks of completion of therapy.

Diagnosis

Diagnosis of CDI requires the presence of diarrhea (at least 3 unformed stools in 24 hours) or radiographic evidence of ileus or toxic megacolon, in addition to positive stool testing for *C. difficile* toxin or colonoscopic or pathologic findings showing pseudomembranes [9].

It is important to limit stool testing to patients with significant diarrhea, since colonization with *C. difficile* is relatively common [6].

The stool cytotoxicity (CTA) and the toxigenic culture (TC) methods had been used in the diagnosis of CDI. The CTA is sensitive and specific but it is relatively slow, time-consuming and expensive for the necessity of maintaining cell lines. For regards the TC, it is either very slow (48 to 72 hours) or laborious. Moreover, the test is not able to identify the non-toxigenic strains. Therefore both conventional methods are unlikely to be adopted by a clinical laboratory as the standard methods for *C. difficile* testing. As of today, most laboratories have adopted enzyme immunoassays (EIAs) for toxins A and B as the routine method of testing [7].

The diagnosis of CDI recommends the use of a two or three-step algorithm. The first step consists of either a glutamate dehydrogenase enzyme immunoassay (GDH-EIA) or the nucleic acid amplification test (NAATs) as screening test. Samples resulting negative from the first step can be reported as negative CDI, but those with positive results should be confirmed (toxins-EIA). Subsequently, the samples confirmed by this second step can be reported as positive CDI [7].

GDH-EIA
C. difficile produces and secretes GDH, which allows to the bacterium to limit the oxidative stress derived from inactivating hydrogen peroxide through the production of ketoglutarate. Several studies have shown a sensitivity of 85-95% and a specificity of 89-99%, underlining in particular a high negative predictive value, making it useful for a rapid screening. However, its value is limited because it is not able to discriminate between toxigenic and non-toxigenic strains [7].

NAATs
NAATs detect one or more specific genes of toxigenic strains; the critical gene is *tcdB*, which encodes for toxin B. NAATs are highly sensitive compared to EIA. NAATs are specific for toxigenic strains but do not test for active toxin protein production. Moreover, NAATs are capable of detecting asymptomatic

carriers of *C. difficile* leading to either an overdiagnosis of CDI or an antibiotic treatment of patients who may not require such therapy with subsequently overestimation of hospital CDI rates. For circumstances in which initial testing consisted of NAAT (with positive result) is appropriate subsequent testing with the toxins EIA to bolster the clinical specificity [7].

Toxin - EIA

Although some strains produce only toxin B, most *C. difficile* strains produce both toxins A and B. No CDI due to strains producing toxin A alone has been reported. In the last two decades, the toxins EIA has been among the most widely used for diagnosing CDI for their rapid and inexpensive performance despite their poor sensitivity (around 60%). This assay shows a better specificity (up to 99%). Moreover, it is important to note that *C. difficile* toxin degrades at room temperature and might be undetectable within two hours after collection; therefore, specimens should be kept at 4°C. To overcome these limits, the NAATs represent the best method to detect the toxigenic strains [7].

Severity Criteria

Severity criteria for *C. difficile* infection are defined by the European Society of Clinical Microbiology and Infectious Diseases (ESCMID) [10]:

- Physical examination:
  - Fever (core body temperature > 38.5°C).
  - Rigors (uncontrollable shaking and a feeling of cold followed by a rise in body temperature).
  - Haemodynamic instability including signs of distributive shock.
  - Respiratory failure requiring mechanical ventilation.
  - Signs and symptoms of peritonitis.
  - Signs and symptoms of colonic ileus.
  - Admixture of blood with stools is rare in *C. difficile* infection and the correlation with severity of disease is uncertain.
- Laboratory investigations:
  - Marked leucocytosis (leucocyte count > 15 x 10^9/L).
  - Marked left shift (band neutrophils > 20% of leucocytes).
  - Rise in serum creatinine (>50% above baseline).

- Elevated serum lactate (≥5 mM).
- Markedly reduced serum albumin (<30 g/L).
- Colonoscopy or sigmoidoscopy:
  - Pseudomembranous colitis.
  - There is insufficient knowledge on the correlation of endoscopic findings compatible with CDI, such as edema, erythema, friability and ulceration, and the severity of disease.
- Imaging:
  - Distension of large intestine (>6 cm in transverse width of colon).
  - Colonic wall thickening, including low-attenuation mural thickening.
  - Pericolonic fat stranding.
  - Ascites not explained by other causes.
  - The correlation of haustral or mucosal thickening, including thumbprinting, pseudopolyps and plaques, with severity of disease is unclear.

Treatment

Medical Treatment

Treatment of CDI involves discontinuation of the offending antibiotic, whenever possible. Antiperistaltic agents should be avoided, at least until antibiotic therapy is well underway [6].

Until recently, the antibiotics metronidazole and vancomycin were the only pharmacological options for the treatment of CDI. Metronidazole may be administered orally or intravenously, whereas vancomycin may be given orally or per rectum for this indication. Vancomycin is not used intravenously to treat CDI because it has very limited penetration into the gut mucosa [3].

The treatment depends on the severity of the disease [8]. Metronidazole is the drug of choice for mild infection (500 mg by mouth three times a day for 10-14 days), while vancomycin should be used for more severe episodes (125 mg by mouth four times daily for 10-14 days). Recurrence rates over 30% have been reported [6].

Mild-to-Moderate Disease

Metronidazole 500 mg orally three times a day for 10 days. If unable to take metronidazole, vancomycin 125 mg orally four times a day for 10 days. If no improvement in 5-7 days, consider change to vancomycin at standard dose (vancomycin 125 mg four times a day for 10 days) [8].

Severe Disease
Vancomycin 125 mg orally four times a day for 10 days [8].

Severe and Complicated Disease
Vancomycin 500 mg orally four times a day and metronidazole 500 mg IV every 8 hours, and vancomycin per rectum (vancomycin 500 mg in 500 ml saline as enema) four times a day. Surgical consultation is suggested [8].

Recurrent CDI
Repeat metronidazole or vancomycin pulse regimen. Consider fecal microbiota transplant after 3 recurrences [8].

Teicoplanin and tigecycline can be effective in the treatment of the severe CDI [4]. On the other hand, Fidaxomicin is a novel macrocyclic antibiotic, which is more active against NAP1/BI/027 strains and it is administered orally in order to treat recurrent CDI [3, 6].

Fecal Microbiota Transplantation
Fecal microbiota transplantation has typically been reserved for patients who have refractory *C. difficile* colitis [3]. It should be considered after 3 recurrences [8].

Surgical Treatment
When medical therapy fails in patients with complicated CDI surgical consultation should be obtained. Surgical therapy should be considered in patients with any one of the following attributed to CDI: hypotension requiring vasopressor therapy, clinical signs of sepsis and organ dysfunction (renal and pulmonary), mental status changes, WBC count $\geq$ 50,000 cells/µl, lactate $\geq$ 5 mmol/l or failure to improve on medical therapy after 5 days [6, 8].

Abdominal colectomy is the treatment of choice for severely ill patients. Patients with megacolon, perforation or an acute abdomen should have an emergency colectomy [6].

Infection Control and Prevention

Rifaximin is a non-absorbable rifamycin antibiotic that has been tested to prevent recurrences after completion of standard antibiotic therapy [4].

Probiotics are live microorganisms administered to restore a dysbiotic environment and potentially prevent *C. difficile* infection [4]. Single and small combination probiotic agents have shown modest success in risk reduction of CDI in high-risk patients receiving systemic antibiotics [11].

Recommendations for the control and prevention of outbreaks of CDI are described below [8]:

- A hospital-based infection control program can help to decrease the incidence of CDI.
- Routine screening for *C. difficile* in hospitalized patients without diarrhea is not recommended and asymptomatic carriers should not be treated.
- Restriction of the most common off ending antimicrobials is effective in CDI prevention.
- Contact precautions for a patient with CDI should be maintained at a minimum until the resolution of diarrhea.
- Patients with known or suspected CDI should be placed in a private room or in a room with another patient with documented CDI.
- Hand hygiene and barrier precautions, including gloves and gowns, should be used by all health-care workers and visitors entering the room of any patient with known or suspected CDI.
- Single-use disposable equipment should be used for prevention of CDI transmission. Non-disposable medical equipment should be dedicated to the patient's room, and other equipment should be thoroughly cleaned after use in a patient with CDI.
- Disinfection of environmental surfaces is recommended using an Environmental Protection Agency (EPA) registered disinfectant with *C. difficile* sporicidal label claim or 5000 p.p.m. chlorinecontaining cleaning agents in areas of potential contamination by *C. difficile*.
- Although there is moderate evidence that two probiotics (*L. rhamnosus* GG and *S. boulardii*) decrease the incidence of antibiotics-associated diarrhea, there is insufficient evidence that probiotics prevent CDI.

Conclusion

Antibiotics-associated diarrhea affects 5-39% of people treated with antibiotics and it is estimated that *C. difficile* is implicated in 10-25% of cases. In turn, it is calculated that 75% of antibiotic-associated colitis cases are caused by C. *difficile*, and of those, 90-100% are pseudomembranous colitis. Diagnosis of CDI requires the presence of diarrhea (at least 3 unformed stools in 24 hours) or radiographic evidence of ileus or toxic megacolon, in addition to positive stool testing for *C. difficile* toxin or colonoscopic or pathologic findings showing pseudomembranes. Treatment of CDI involves discontinuation of the offending antibiotic, whenever possible. The antibiotics metronidazole and vancomycin are the main pharmacological options for the treatment of CDI. Single and small combination probiotic agents have shown modest success in risk reduction of CDI in high-risk patients receiving systemic antibiotics.

References

[1] Bouza E. Consequences of *Clostridium difficile* infection: understanding the healthcare burden. *Clin Microbiol Infect.* 2012;18 Suppl 6:5-12.
[2] Del Prete R., Ronga L., Addati G., Magrone R., Abbasciano A., Decimo M., Miragliotta G. *Clostridium difficile*. A review on an emerging infection. *Clin Ter.* 2019 Jan-Feb;170(1):e41-e47.
[3] Mullish B. H., Williams H. R. *Clostridium difficile* infection and antibiotic-associated diarrhoea. *Clin Med* (Lond). 2018 Jun;18(3):237-241.
[4] Guery B., Galperine T., Barbut F. *Clostridioides difficile*: diagnosis and treatments. *BMJ.* 2019;366:l4609.
[5] Alyousef A. A. *Clostridium difficile*: Epidemiology, Pathogenicity, and an Update on the Limitations of and Challenges in Its Diagnosis. *J AOAC Int.* 2018;101:1119-26.
[6] Ong G. K., Reidy T. J., Huk M. D., Lane F. R. *Clostridium difficile* colitis: A clinical review. *Am J Surg.* 2017;213:565-71.
[7] Del Prete R., Ronga L., Addati G., Magrone R., Abbasciano A., Decimo M., et al., *Clostridium difficile*. A review on an emerging infection. *Clin Ter.* 2019;170:e41-e47.
[8] Surawicz C. M., Brandt L. J., Binion D. G., Ananthakrishnan A. N., Curry S. R., Gilligan P. H., McFarland L. V., Mellow M., Zuckerbraun B. S. Guidelines for diagnosis, treatment, and prevention of *Clostridium difficile* infections. *Am J Gastroenterol.* 2013;108:478-98.

[9] Cohen S. H., Gerding D. N., Johnson S., et al., Clinical practice guidelines for *Clostridium difficile* infection in adults: 2010 update by the society for healthcare epidemiology of America (SHEA) and the infectious diseases society of America (IDSA). *Infect Cont Hosp Ep*. 2010;31:431e455.

[10] Debast S. B., Bauer M. P., Kuijper E. J., European Society of Clinical Microbiology and Infectious Diseases. European Society of Clinical Microbiology and Infectious Diseases: update of the treatment guidance document for *Clostridium difficile* infection. *Clin Microbiol Infect*. 2014;20(Suppl 2):1-26.

[11] Mills J. P., Rao K., Young V. B. Probiotics for prevention of *Clostridium difficile* infection. *Curr Opin Gastroenterol*. 2018;34:3-10.

Editors' Contact Information

Jaime Ruiz-Tovar, MD, PhD
Professor of Surgery,
Universidad Alfonso X,
Virgen da la Oliva, Madrid, Spain
jruiztovar@gmail.com

Andrés García Marín, PhD
Department of Surgery,
Hospital de Hellin, Albacete, Spain
Professor of Surgery,
Universidad Alfonso X,
Virgen da la Oliva, Madrid, Spain
agmarin1980@gmail.com

Index

A

abdominal surgery, v, vii, 7, 8, 9, 10, 13, 19, 29, 31, 59, 62
access, 8, 23, 74, 78, 84, 85, 98, 102
acute respiratory distress syndrome, 11, 61, 64
adults, 5, 10, 14, 54, 58, 68, 69, 88, 100, 113
adverse effects, 25, 86
antibiotic, vii, 4, 8, 12, 13, 15, 20, 25, 36, 37, 38, 39, 41, 42, 52, 56, 59, 60, 62, 63, 64, 65, 66, 67, 68, 70, 80, 82, 84, 85, 86, 87, 93, 94, 95, 96, 98, 99, 100, 104, 105, 108, 109, 110, 111, 112
antibiotic ointment, 84
antibiotic resistance, 65, 86
antimicrobial therapy, 38, 42, 45, 57, 60, 73, 85
aseptic, 55, 82, 83, 84, 87, 97, 100
aspiration, 8, 23, 61, 62, 64, 65, 70, 71
asymptomatic, 56, 107, 111
atmospheric pressure, 28

B

bacteremia, 2, 3, 4, 5, 10, 13, 50, 55, 60, 74, 75, 78, 79, 80, 81, 85, 87, 88, 94, 97, 98, 99, 100
bacteria, 20, 23, 27, 28, 37, 41, 45, 49, 51, 56, 57, 64, 66, 71, 73, 78, 82, 85, 86, 87, 92, 94, 96, 104
bacterial infection, 11, 15
bacterial pathogens, 61
bacterium, 53, 107

blood cultures, 2, 73, 80, 81, 82, 94, 95, 96, 98, 99
blood flow, 28
blood stream, 70, 87
blood transfusion, 15, 17, 66
blood transfusions, 66
bloodstream, 5, 8, 16, 36, 73, 74, 81, 87, 88, 102
body fluid, 13
bone marrow, 76
bone marrow transplant, 76

C

cardiac risk, 12
cardiac risk factors, 12
cardiac surgery, 14, 70, 93
catheter, vii, 3, 4, 5, 16, 36, 45, 46, 47, 48, 49, 50, 51, 53, 54, 55, 57, 58, 64, 73, 74, 75, 76, 77, 78, 79, 80, 81, 82, 83, 84, 85, 86, 87, 88, 89, 97, 98, 99, 100, 101, 102
catheter-associated urinary tract infections, 36, 45, 46, 57, 58
catheter-related bloodstream infections, 16, 73, 74, 87, 102
cefazolin, 25, 32, 56, 86, 99
cephalosporin, 42, 56, 85
chemotherapy, 2, 60, 75, 76
clinical presentation, 50
clinical trials, 10, 24, 26
clostridium difficile, 3, 5, 36, 37, 103, 104, 112, 113
colonization, 11, 28, 33, 38, 39, 47, 48, 49, 61, 62, 73, 77, 81, 82, 98, 107

Index

community, 2, 3, 5, 36, 38, 42, 47, 56, 95, 104
complications, vii, 9, 11, 21, 28, 55, 66, 79, 80, 81, 83, 86, 92, 94, 95, 96, 99
congenital heart disease, 92
congestive heart failure, 63
contamination, vii, 20, 21, 27, 28, 29, 30, 38, 51, 77, 78, 79, 111
cost, 21, 31, 45, 46, 54, 66, 69, 73
cost effectiveness, 31
culture, 51, 52, 53, 56, 64, 67, 70, 80, 81, 82, 94, 95, 99, 107

D

developed countries, 3, 5, 91, 104
diabetes, 7, 11, 28, 38, 48
diabetic patients, 10, 16
diagnostic criteria, 63, 94
diarrhea, 3, 5, 104, 106, 107, 111, 112
diseases, 2, 46, 48, 58, 113
drainage, 13, 25, 37, 48, 49, 55, 71, 79
drugs, viii, 8, 35, 37, 41, 42, 56, 58, 96
dysuria, 45, 50, 52, 53, 56, 57

E

edema, vii, 28, 109
emboli, 61, 79, 98
embolization, 61, 98
emergency, vii, 12, 95, 97, 110
endocrine disorders, 12
endotracheal intubation, 60, 62, 65, 68
environmental contamination, 16
epidemiology, 1, 5, 16, 41, 46, 103, 113
equipment, 36, 49, 61, 111
erythrocyte sedimentation rate, 93
evidence, vii, viii, 1, 23, 24, 25, 27, 30, 31, 52, 54, 64, 69, 85, 103, 107, 111, 112
extracellular matrix, 49

F

false negative, 64
false positive, 63
fever, 45, 50, 52, 53, 56, 63, 73, 79, 80, 88, 93, 94, 106
flora, 4, 8, 20, 29, 49, 50, 104

fluid, 12, 14, 28, 35, 37, 41, 71
fluoroquinolones, 56, 105
formation, 28, 49, 50, 55, 86, 105
fungal infection, 61
fungi, 35, 37, 41, 92, 96

G

gastroesophageal reflux, 65
gastrointestinal tract, 61
general anesthesia, 7, 11
genitourinary tract, vii, 92
glucose, 10, 14, 15, 16, 79
growth, 29, 45, 49, 51, 67
guidelines, vii, 16, 19, 26, 30, 31, 32, 38, 54, 58, 68, 82, 88, 89, 95, 101, 113

H

health, vii, 2, 4, 5, 8, 20, 30, 37, 52, 57, 71, 78, 111
health care, 2, 5, 37, 57, 78
healthcare-acquired infection, 36
heart disease, 38, 93
heart failure, 96
heart murmur, 93
heart valves, 80, 91
hemodialysis, 2, 60, 74, 75, 76, 78, 84, 86
hemodynamic instability, 73
hospital acquired infections, 74
hospital-acquired infection, 35, 36, 41, 45, 46, 57, 73
hospitalization, 3, 12, 37, 61, 62
hydrogen peroxide, 107
hygiene, 13, 82, 87, 97, 111

I

identification, 63, 94, 95
immune function, 10, 11
immune response, 15, 21, 105
immune system, vii, 8, 21, 48
immunosuppression, 7, 11, 25, 36, 39, 48, 98
impact, 1, 2, 3, 15, 17, 26, 33, 41, 43, 70, 88, 103, 104

Index

incidence, 1, 3, 4, 5, 9, 14, 20, 21, 22, 24, 26, 27, 29, 33, 55, 58, 59, 60, 63, 65, 66, 69, 74, 76, 91, 92, 97, 100, 104, 111
infection, v, vii, 1, 2, 3, 4, 5, 7, 8, 9, 10, 11, 12, 13, 14, 15, 16, 19, 20, 28, 30, 31, 32, 33, 35, 36, 38, 41, 42, 43, 45, 46, 47, 53, 55, 56, 57, 58, 59, 60, 61, 62, 63, 64, 66, 67, 70, 71, 73, 74, 75, 76, 77, 78, 79, 80, 81, 82, 83, 84, 85, 87, 88, 89, 91, 93, 96, 97, 98, 99, 100, 101, 102, 103, 104, 105, 108, 109, 111, 112, 113
infection etiology, 1
infective endocarditis (IE), 79, 80, 91, 92, 93, 94, 95, 96, 99, 100, 101
inflammation, 10, 38, 49, 73, 79, 104
inflammatory cells, 91
initiation, 9, 38, 39, 59, 80, 82
insertion, vii, 13, 49, 55, 73, 74, 77, 79, 80, 82, 83, 84, 87, 88, 93, 97, 98, 100
insulin, 10, 15, 23, 31
insulin resistance, 10
insulin sensitivity, 23
intensive care unit, 5, 37, 41, 42, 70, 97, 106
intervention, 16, 21, 23, 38, 102
intestinal tract, 49, 66
intravascular infections, v, 91, 97, 98
intravenous antibiotics, 61
intravenous fluids, 74, 75

L

laboratory tests, 80
laparoscopic cholecystectomy, 25, 32
leukocytes, 51, 52, 64, 76
leukocytosis, 63, 94
liver, 11, 37, 39, 40
liver cirrhosis, 11
liver disease, 37

M

management, 13, 21, 32, 38, 39, 41, 42, 46, 47, 54, 58, 65, 66, 68, 69, 71, 84, 87, 89, 92, 94, 98, 99, 100, 101, 103, 104
manipulation, 92, 93

mechanical ventilation, 4, 5, 8, 60, 62, 65, 68, 71, 106, 108
medical, viii, 55, 60, 77, 110, 111
medication, 12, 13, 74, 75
mental status changes, 110
meta-analysis, 9, 11, 12, 14, 15, 24, 26, 31, 60, 64, 70, 71, 101
microbiology, v, 35, 36, 37, 46, 52, 58, 78, 88, 101, 108, 113
microorganism, 4, 11, 20, 35, 49, 61, 81, 98
microorganisms, vii, 4, 8, 20, 24, 25, 29, 37, 38, 41, 45, 47, 49, 50, 51, 57, 61, 73, 78, 81, 91, 92, 96, 99, 111
morbidity, vii, 12, 15, 21, 45, 46, 54, 59, 60, 69, 73, 76, 100
mortality, vii, 3, 5, 10, 12, 15, 16, 17, 21, 36, 38, 42, 43, 45, 46, 54, 59, 60, 62, 63, 66, 69, 70, 73, 76, 87, 92, 95, 99, 100
mortality rate, 38, 92, 95
mucosa, 92, 109
multidrug- resistant pathogens, 36
multivariate analysis, 68
musculoskeletal, 79, 80, 92

N

nosocomial infection, v, vii, 1, 2, 3, 4, 5, 7, 8, 9, 10, 11, 12, 13, 14, 16, 20, 35, 36, 41, 45, 46, 58, 59, 60, 73, 74, 103
nosocomial pneumonia, 9, 59, 63
nosocomial site infection, v, 35, 36
nutrition, 9, 14, 15, 16, 21, 22, 23, 31, 38, 74, 75, 79, 86
nutritional status, 12, 20, 21, 22, 23

O

obesity, 14, 15, 20
organ, 8, 9, 10, 20, 37, 38, 65, 106, 110
organism, 55, 93, 95
oxygen, 11, 14, 15, 28, 49, 64

P

pain, 50, 52, 53, 56, 80, 106
pathogenesis, viii, 46, 49, 103, 105

Index

pathogens, 13, 20, 35, 36, 37, 38, 41, 45, 49, 50, 57, 59, 61, 62, 63, 66, 85, 96
pathology, 12, 48, 91
peripheral blood, 81, 98
peritonitis, 29, 42, 43, 108
phlebitis, 97, 99, 100
pneumonia, 3, 4, 5, 8, 9, 10, 13, 36, 59, 60, 62, 63, 66, 68, 69, 70, 71, 79
preparation, iv, vii, 13, 24, 26, 32
prevention, vii, 3, 4, 5, 7, 12, 13, 15, 19, 28, 30, 31, 32, 36, 41, 43, 45, 46, 52, 54, 57, 58, 63, 65, 70, 71, 73, 74, 76, 82, 84, 87, 88, 91, 92, 96, 97, 100, 103, 111, 112, 113
prognosis, 13, 42, 62, 68, 95
proliferation, 91, 99
prophylactic, viii, 65
prophylaxis, 12, 13, 15, 19, 25, 31, 32, 55, 65, 92, 93, 99, 100
pseudomembranous colitis, v, 103, 104, 109, 112
Pseudomonas aeruginosa, 35, 37, 38, 41, 50, 59, 60, 61, 67
pulmonary artery, 75
pulmonary embolism, 63
pyelonephritis, 46, 47, 57
pyuria, 45, 51, 52, 56, 57

Q

quality of life, vii, 21, 31, 85

R

recommendations, iv, vii, 19, 21, 26, 27, 29, 30, 66, 71, 82, 87
renal replacement therapy, 61
resistance, 24, 42, 55, 56, 67, 74, 76, 79, 84, 98
respiratory distress syndrome, 62
respiratory dysfunction, 61
respiratory infections, 9, 59
response, 28, 38, 56, 66, 67, 68, 105
risk factors, v, 1, 7, 9, 10, 11, 12, 13, 14, 28, 38, 45, 46, 47, 48, 50, 54, 56, 57, 59, 61, 62, 66, 69, 73, 76, 87, 97, 101, 103, 105

S

sensitivity, 63, 94, 96, 107, 108
sepsis, 12, 14, 16, 21, 38, 39, 41, 88, 98, 100, 110
signs, 38, 50, 51, 53, 63, 80, 87, 94, 96, 97, 98, 99, 100, 106, 108, 110
skin, 12, 13, 20, 23, 24, 26, 27, 28, 29, 30, 31, 73, 75, 76, 77, 78, 81, 82, 84
species, 52, 53, 60, 92, 98, 99
staphylococci, 4, 20, 37, 41, 61, 73, 78, 82, 93, 95, 96, 98
sterile, 24, 47, 51, 55, 84, 97
subcutaneous tissue, 15, 29, 30
surgical site infection, v, vii, 3, 4, 8, 9, 12, 14, 15, 19, 28, 30, 31, 32, 33, 35, 36, 41, 43, 46, 47
surgical site infections, 19, 28, 31, 32, 36, 43, 46, 47
susceptibility, 37, 38, 41, 56, 67, 76, 94
symptoms, 47, 50, 51, 52, 53, 56, 63, 79, 80, 93, 96, 106, 108

T

techniques, vii, 2, 64, 82, 83, 87, 94
temperature, 14, 27, 108
testing, 94, 107, 108, 112
therapy, 15, 25, 28, 31, 32, 33, 36, 38, 39, 42, 45, 56, 57, 59, 60, 66, 68, 70, 79, 80, 82, 84, 85, 86, 87, 95, 99, 106, 108, 109, 110, 111
tissue, vii, 11, 12, 14, 25, 76, 81, 95
tissue perfusion, 12
toxin, 104, 105, 107, 108, 112
trauma, 8, 11, 14, 33, 62, 69, 76
treatment, v, vii, 2, 8, 10, 11, 12, 28, 35, 36, 37, 39, 42, 43, 46, 51, 52, 54, 55, 56, 58, 59, 62, 63, 64, 65, 66, 67, 68, 74, 82, 83, 84, 85, 86, 87, 88, 91, 93, 95, 96, 98, 99, 103, 104, 108, 109, 110, 112, 113

U

urinary bladder, 48
urinary tract, 3, 4, 5, 8, 9, 13, 36, 45, 46, 47, 48, 54, 55, 56, 57, 58, 81

urinary tract infection, 3, 4, 5, 8, 9, 13, 36, 45, 46, 55, 56, 57, 58
urinary tract infections, 3, 4, 8, 9, 13, 45, 46, 56, 57, 58
urine, 45, 49, 51, 52, 53, 56

V

valvular heart disease, 101
vancomycin, 25, 36, 38, 57, 67, 85, 86, 99, 109, 110, 112
vascular access infections, 74
vegetation, 91, 94, 96

vein, 74, 75, 82, 98, 99
ventilation, 12, 60, 65, 68
vitamin D, 36, 41

W

worldwide, 45, 46, 73, 76, 104
wound dehiscence, 28
wound healing, 13, 21
wound infection, 10, 11, 24